The Student Nurse
Handbook

For Baillière Tindall:

Senior Commissioning Editor: Ninette Premdas
Project Development Manager: Katrina Mather
Project Manager: Joannah Duncan
Design: Judith Wright

The Student Nurse Handbook

A Survival Guide

Bethann Siviter BSc(Hons) RN(Adult) DNCert Dip(HE)
Past Chair of the RCN Association of Nursing Students
District Nurse Team Leader, Rowley Regis & Tipton PCT, UK

With a contribution from:
Denise Stevens RCN(Learning Disability) Dip(HE)
Learning disability nurse

Foreword by:
Jonathan Asbridge
President, NMC, London, UK

Edinburgh • London • New York • Philadelphia • St Louis • Sydney • Toronto 2004

BAILLIÈRE TINDALL
An imprint of Elsevier Limited

First published 2004

ISBN 0 7020 2730 8

British Library Cataloguing in Publication Data
A catalogue record for this book is available from the British Library

Library of Congress Cataloging in Publication Data
A catalog record for this book is available from the Library of Congress

Note
Medical knowledge is constantly changing. As new information becomes available, changes in treatment, procedures, equipment and the use of drugs become necessary. The author, contributors and the publishers have taken care to ensure that the information given in this text is accurate and up to date. However, readers are strongly advised to confirm that the information, especially with regard to drug usage, complies with the latest legislation and standards of practice.

your source for books,
journals and multimedia
in the health sciences
www.elsevierhealth.com

The
Publisher's
policy is to use
**paper manufactured
from sustainable forests**

Printed in China

Contents

To Fiona Malem
Nurse, mentor, teacher, friend, inspiration.

Acknowledgements

I need to thank a few people:

Fiona Malem
Dorothy Vaitkunas, my mom and first role model in nursing
Judy Gerrard and Elaine Elwell
Jane Gardiner
Sue Hinchliff
Roger Cobley
Debbie Dandy
George Castledine
Executive Committee and RCN Council

and, most importantly, a sincere and humble thank you to my husband Andrew Siviter, without whose support, love, constant encouragement, enduring patience (and not inconsiderable overdraft) I could not have survived my course, my work as an advocate, or written this book. He deserves all the credit for anything I manage to accomplish.

Relationships can take a real beating when you are in nurse education – don't forget to let your partners, friends and children know how much you appreciate them for helping you get through. I don't think I could ever thank my husband enough. There have been so many people – at the University of Central England (UCE), at Heartlands Hospital, at Great Bridge Partnerships for Health and Regent Street Medical Centre, at Selly Oak and Queen Elizabeth Hospitals, at University of Wolverhampton, at the Birmingham and the Black Country Workforce Planning Confederation and The Birmingham and the Black Country Strategic Health Authority, at Rowley Regis & Tipton PCT, Smethwick & Oldbury PCT, and West Bromwich & Wednesbury PCT, and especially the Royal College of Nursing (RCN), RCN Council, the RCN Association of Nursing Students (ANS) and the ANS Executive Committee – who have helped and supported me that I can't name them all, but I hope they know how very grateful I am. I hope this book can serve to give you a little of the help and support these wonderful people have given me.

Foreword

As President of the NMC (Nursing and Midwifery Council) and as a nurse I am strongly committed to supporting student nurses. I know I share this belief with the author. Bethann has been a passionate activist on behalf of United Kingdom student nurses; it is obvious throughout the text that it is her goal to provide, in a personal and direct way, information and advice that only one who has recently been through the student experience can impart. Her recent qualification and involvement as a national level activist gives her credibility and sensitivity to the challenges students and prospective students have ahead of them.

Although the student nurse is not accountable for their practice, under the Nursing and Midwifery Council (NMC) Code of Professional Conduct (2002), during their pre-registration education, it is essential that the student nurse develops the skills, knowledge and insight necessary to be a competent and accountable qualified nurse. This book establishes a foundation from which student nurses can develop accountability and ownership for their professional development and practice. It is, however, not a clinical textbook, it is a practical survival guide which uses common sense and humour to make important points.

The Student Nurse Handbook gives the student advice about academic preparation and clinical placements, and challenges the nursing student to develop insight into themselves and their eventual role in nursing. It encourages the student to embrace the role of patient advocate. It also gives hints and advice that many student nurses might only discover through trial and error: it should prevent considerable frustration and stress. It also provides the full text of key NMC documents and encourages students to become familiar with and regularly use these resources. The NMC is not simply a regulatory body, but a valuable source of professional information and support. An essential part of the NMC mandate to protect the public is helping nurses prepare for and maintain competent practice. Remember throughout your education and career that the NMC is there for you.

This book is an unique and invaluable resource which you will find useful throughout your days as a student and during your career as a nurse. I'd like to congratulate Bethann Siviter on this book. And as a final note, I would like to welcome you to the world of nursing, and re-assure you that we as a community of nurses eagerly await your arrival.

Jonathan Asbridge
UK 2004

Preface

I want to tell you why I think I have the right to write this book. It is important for you to know a bit about me so you know you can trust what I am telling you.

Before moving to England, I was a Licensed Practical Nurse in America. My nursing programme there was a traditional 'in-hospital' course where I studied, complete with nurse's hat and a quaking fear of the school's director. As a nurse in America I worked in acute and long-term care and in the community. Despite being a nurse for a number of years, I had to start from the beginning in nursing when I moved to England and I studied for my Diploma in Adult Nursing at the University of Central England (UCE) in Birmingham.

My placements were in hospitals and clinical settings around Birmingham. I had some very good placements and a few very bad ones. My first placement nearly drove me out of nursing it was so terrible, and my last one was so wonderful that I nearly took a job on that unit.

It was while I was at UCE that I was approached about becoming active as a student activist in the Royal College of Nursing (RCN). Because of my nursing background in America and my status as a 'mature' student, Fiona "Mrs Mayhem" Malem (a senior lecturer and student advocate) took me under her wing. She was a real inspiration and, among other things, taught me:

> If you are the one to see the problem,
> then you are the one who should try and fix it...

I have dedicated this book to Fiona because of her caring, her wisdom, her inspiration and her love. It's my great sadness that she is not here to see this book: it is because of her that it was written. I hope each one of you has lecturers and mentors like Fiona.

While completing my diploma, I became a student steward, then a member of the RCN's Association of Nursing Students Executive Committee as representative for the West Midlands. I was elected as Student Member to the RCN's Council and then as Chair of the Association of Nursing Students. During all this, I was studying, attending placements, always running late for my bus, carrying as many books as they would let me take from the library, killing a few pints in the student union bar with my friends, worrying about my overdraft and staying up until the wee hours to get assignments done. Sound familiar?

In addition to my own experiences, as a national level student activist I have heard student nurses from all over the UK talking about their problems and their fears – and students from Belfast to Birmingham and from Barra to Bangor all say the same kinds of things. They desperately want to be good nurses, are struggling with hardship and with part-time work, feel burdened with academic work, are afraid they will not have the skills and knowledge they need, and – despite being stressed, worried and tired – they care deeply for their patients and want to do the best for them that they can.

That's why I wanted to write this book. I hope that it will become a friend for you, a place where you can look for information when you are stuck, where you can find guidance, perhaps some inspiration, a little information and the reassurance that you *can* do it. I've tried to make it light but with serious points, and kept it very honest and direct. This book is the book that I wished I could have found when I was on my course. If you think there are things that don't belong here, or have suggestions to make anything better, please let me know. This book is for you and I want it to be useful no matter which branch or country you are in. I'd love to hear from you and know how you are getting on.

One other thing – I personally have been very active in the Royal College of Nursing. I know colleagues who have received tremendous support from Unison and from other unions. When I refer to your 'union rep', I mean the rep from whichever union you decide is best for you. It's not up to me to tell you which one that is: they all have good and bad points. But *please* join a union – they don't charge students very much and are an important source of information and support.

Bethann Siviter

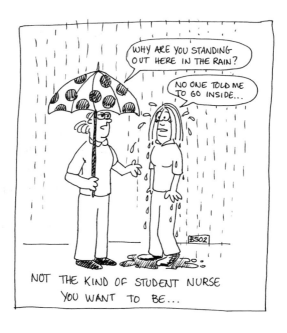

NOT THE KIND OF STUDENT NURSE YOU WANT TO BE...

Nursing and Nurse Education

❝ I always wanted to be a nurse, but my mother was a nurse, so I thought maybe I was doing it just to be like her. I did everything else – McDonalds, a shop assistant, being a carer – but finally at 31 I found myself becoming a nurse anyway ... ❞

Newly qualified nurse

❝ Everyone said not to become a nurse. The hours and pay scared off a lot of my mates. I couldn't *not* become a nurse, it's what I always wanted to do. The pay and hours are better than people think, and I love my job. As a nurse, I can work anywhere and do anything. Nursing is great. ❞

Newly qualified nurse

In this chapter

> *Just a note*
>
> 'Uni' or 'university': when discussing the institutions where nursing students prepare to become nurses, I refer to universities or unis. This isn't meant to discount non-university courses in smaller schools or colleges of nursing that are not in university per se – it's for ease in explaining. When you read 'uni' or 'university', just know I mean all kinds of nurse education programmes.
>
>   'Student Grants Unit': although the Student Grants Unit is specifically for students based in England, most countries have an equivalent; Check the list of contacts at the end of this chapter. When I refer to the Student Grants Unit I mean whichever one is relevant to you.

WHAT IS NURSING?

To quote TS Eliot's poem *The ad-dressing of cats:*

> ‘ A dog's a dog – but a cat's a CAT!
>   A cat is not a dog … ’

First, let me tell you what nursing is not. Nursing is not the profession you enter when you are not good enough to become a medic, or when your grades aren't good enough for other courses of study. It's not 'just women's work'. It's not the way to get into other careers or professions. It's not the job for someone who just wants to serve (or meet and marry) a member of another profession. It's not a job that you will leave behind you when you go home for the day; it's not the uniform you put on for work.

Nursing is a profession in its own right, with its own history, its own theories and frameworks and its own way of looking at the world. Nursing is something that will become part of you, will guide the way you think and act in every situation, not just at work. Some people jokingly say that becoming a nurse is a terminal disease – it will be there, a part of you, until you are no more.

The way you see the world, and the people in it, will be coloured by your nursing knowledge and judgement.

So stepping into nursing is not just entering a profession – it's allowing the profession to enter you. You might leave nursing and have other careers but what you learn as a nurse will always be a part of you.

Nursing is ...

In 1966, Virginia Henderson, a nursing theorist, wrote:

❛ Nursing is primarily assisting the individual in their performance of those activities contributing to health, or its recovery that they would perform unaided if they had the necessary strength, will, or knowledge. ❜

The Royal College of Nursing (2003) has defined nursing as:

❛ The use of clinical judgement in the provision of care to enable people to improve, maintain, or recover health, to cope with health problems, and to achieve the best possible quality of life, whatever their disease or disability, until death. ❜

Looking at these we see that nurses:

- use clinical judgement, which requires education and experience
- help people who are well stay well
- help people who are ill get better
- help people who won't get better to have the best life possible
- do for people what they would do for themselves
- promote good health
- provide care and services
- help people to cope with problems and concerns
- help many different people of different ages with many different problems
- help and support the families and carers of people receiving nursing care.

WHAT KINDS OF JOBS ARE THERE FOR NURSES?

As a nurse, you can work in many different areas and with many different people. There are now four different basic Branches in nursing. During your pre-registration course you can become:

- a children's nurse
- an adult nurse
- a learning disability nurse
- a mental health nurse.

You will need to choose, usually when you apply, which Branch of nursing you want to enter. If you are really unhappy, or find yourself very interested in another Branch, you may be able to change but the sooner you do this the easier it will be.

A nurse can work as a:

- **Midwife:** caring for pregnant women, delivering and caring for their babies. You can become a midwife without being a nurse, or you can take a midwifery course after becoming a nurse. It's a complex and demanding profession that is independent from nursing. If it's really your life desire to become a midwife, apply first to a midwifery course. The transition from nurse to midwife can be difficult for some, as permission to enter the course can be affected by workforce needs, such as a shortage of nurses needed in other areas.

- **Health visitor (HV):** helping new mothers and teaching them how to care for their children, helping those children to be healthy, and/or promoting good health for other groups such as the elderly. Health visitors have an essential role in child protection and work closely with social workers, midwives, learning disability and children's nurses, as well as with other nurses and professionals to maintain good public health and safety for vulnerable children and adults. Becoming a health visitor requires an additional post-basic qualification at degree or postgraduate diploma level. At some point, being a health visitor may become completely independent from a basic nursing qualification.

- **Children's nurse:** a specialist in the health and care of children. A children's nurse can work in any area of care where there are children. Children's nursing is one of the basic pre-registration nursing Branches.
- **Adult nurse:** adult nurses work in the community, in hospitals, in care homes, clinics, etc. Adult nurses are specially prepared for the care and support of people from early adulthood to old age in a variety of settings. Adult nursing is one of the basic pre-registration Branches.
- **Learning disability nurse:** a specialist in caring for and meeting the needs of people with learning disabilities. A learning disability nurse can work in a hospital, care home, school or in a patient's home – wherever there is a client with special needs. Learning disability nursing is one of the basic pre-registration Branches.
- **Mental health nurse:** a nurse specializing in the care and support of people with mental illness. A mental health nurse can work in any setting where there are clients. Mental health nursing is one of the basic pre-registration Branches.
- **School nurse:** promoting health and supporting children in school. Being a school nurse requires a post-basic qualification at postgraduate diploma or degree level.
- **Occupational health nurse:** protecting and caring for people at work. Occupational health nurses do first aid, offer counselling on stress, promote healthy practices at home and at work, and help employers keep their employees healthy. Being an occupational health nurse requires a post-basic qualification at postgraduate diploma or degree level.
- **District nurse:** caring for people in their homes. District nurses have a very broad specialty including wound care, continence and care of chronically ill patients. They work closely with other nurses and other professionals to deliver care and provide support for people who are either too ill or who have such significant mobility problems that they are unable to

easily leave their homes. Being a district nurse requires a post-basic qualification at postgraduate diploma or degree level.

- **Practice nurse (PN):** working in a GP surgery, seeing patients with ongoing problems like asthma or diabetes, doing dressing changes and wound care, giving immunizations and health advice. Practice nurses, like district nurses, work closely with many other nurses and professionals. Being a practice nurse requires a post-basic qualification at postgraduate diploma or degree level.
- **Research nurse:** doing the research to provide evidence for nursing care. Most research nurses will have specialist education and/or a degree.
- **Nurse educator:** teaching both new nurses and nurses learning more advanced practice. Nurse educators come at all different levels. Some nurse educators also continue to work as specialists in their own areas of nursing.
- **Specialist nurse:** specialist nurses work with specific groups of clients, like people with diabetes, cancer, special problems like incontinence or chronic wounds. These specially trained nurses provide support and care for patients and their families while teaching and supporting other nurses. Some nurses, like Marie Curie or MacMillan nurses, are employed by charities to deliver specialist care.
- **Nurse consultant:** nurse consultants are experts who provide care, advice, support and who also work to develop policy and working practices. These nurses usually have a Master's degree level or higher, and have proven expertise in a specific area of nursing.
- **Nurse practitioner:** a highly skilled nurse who delivers an advanced level of care in a certain specialty, such as accident and emergency. These nurses are usually trained at Master's degree level.
- **Prison nurse and forensic nurses:** nurses who work in prisons have a very demanding role – first aid, counselling and health promotion in a strict and sometimes dangerous environment. Prison nurses need both mental health and general nursing

skills. Forensic nurses provide care and ongoing assessment in hospitals, supervised environments and sometimes even in the community where the patient has been convicted of a crime but needs care for a significant mental illness or learning disability. Some forensic nurses have an even wider scope and offer support to victims of crime and trauma as well. Prison and forensic nursing are different but have some similarities, which is why they are listed together.

- **Manager:** a nurse can also work in management, at any one of a number of levels – managing a ward, a specialty area, a clinic, or even nursing at a Trust.
- **Matron:** a matron is a nurse with extensive experience and skill who acts as a supervisor and manager, promoting good practice and supporting the work of other nurses.
- **Community psychiatric nurse:** a mental health nurse who specializes in the care of people in the community. The community psychiatric nurse might visit patients in the hospital, talk to people who are recently bereaved or who have recently suffered an emotional trauma, or may follow clients with mental health needs.
- **Enrolled nurse:** a nurse who is considered to be trained to a lower level than a registered nurse; enrolled nurses typically have to be supervised by a registered nurse. You can no longer become an enrolled nurse in the UK and those who are enrolled nurses are being encouraged to become registered nurses. However, these nurses are skilled and knowledgeable practitioners and are experts in the delivery of hands-on care. Don't underestimate their knowledge and experience.
- **Health care assistant (HCA)/nurse auxilliary (NA):** these caregivers help deliver patient care in nearly every environment in the NHS and healthcare system. Different meanings are sometimes given to the two terms (an NA might be considered to be a higher level than an HCA, or vice versa) and in some places HCAs do more than simply help with nursing tasks (e.g. an HCA in a GP's surgery who also does some clerical work). Many HCAs and NAs are very experienced and have

a wide range of valuable skills. Just because they aren't nurses *per se* doesn't mean that they are not valuable and important members of the healthcare team. In this book, when I refer to HCAs, I mean those in the HCA or NA role.

So, there are as many different kinds of nurses as there are people who need nurses! There is no way I could list every type of nursing – there are countless opportunities for nurses to do work that they enjoy and that interests them.

WHO CAN BECOME A NURSE?

- **Can you listen as well as talk, or are you at least willing to learn?** Much of nursing is less about physical skill and more about communicating and working with people. Your course will help you learn to be a good communicator, so even if you are really shy or quiet you can still learn to become a good nurse.
- **Can you take care of people without being prejudiced or biased?** As a nurse, you will care for criminals, people who abuse drugs or alcohol, people who don't speak English, people who have a different skin colour to yours, elderly and very young people, people with learning disabilities and mental illness, rich people, poor people, likeable people, people who aren't very likeable, clean people, smelly people … and you have to treat them all fairly and with respect.
- **Can you commit to a lifetime of keeping up to date?** Nursing isn't something you learn once and never go back to. Nurses have a commitment to keep their knowledge and skills current.
- **Have you done GCSEs or A levels (or equivalent)?** On the application form, it will explain the minimums. Basically, you need 5 GCSEs or a certain level of national vocational qualification (NVQ). You can find out about the minimum requirements from the Nursing and Midwifery Council (NMC) and from NHS Careers – their contact details are in the Contacts section at the end of this chapter. Some universities want more than the minimum so if you have your heart set on a particular

place, speak to them. Even if you don't have the minimums, you can take the Access course (more on this below). If you are younger than 17 and don't have all the necessary grades you can become a nurse cadet (see below) but nurse cadet schemes run only in England.

- **Do you enjoy being with people?** As a nurse, you will always be with people. But you could be with them in person, over the phone, or in any one of a number of different environments. You could even become a research nurse! No matter how you like to work, there is a place in nursing for you!

- **Are you at least 17?** In Scotland you can start your nurse education at 17; in England, Wales and Northern Ireland you need to be at least 17 and a half when you start your course. Don't worry about being older – the average age of a nursing student is around 30! Many people start their nurse education when their children are older or after they have had a different career.

- **Are you healthy?** Being healthy is important when you are a nurse; you will need to complete a health clearance form when you apply. If you have a disability, don't worry that you can't become a nurse – that's not true. Depending on the disability, you may be able, with the right support, to become a nurse. Ask to talk to the occupational health team when the time comes – don't give up without talking to them first! People with dyslexia, depression and even missing an arm have successfully become nurses.

- **Do you have any criminal convictions?** If you have been convicted of anything, you need to say so on your application form. Most universities ask everyone for a criminal records check anyway, and the university may ask for further information if you do have a problem in your past. They will take the circumstances into consideration, so it's best to be prepared for this and be totally honest about your past when asked. Some types of conviction will make it very difficult to get into nurse education – if you are worried, talk to someone at the university before you apply. Just be totally honest – it's better to show that you learned from your mistakes than have the university think you are dishonest.

As you can see, almost anyone can become a nurse if they really want to. You don't have to be a self-sacrificing angel of mercy to become a good nurse! Even if you don't have a strong academic background, or have had run-ins with the law, or have a disability, you might be able to become a nurse. Contact the groups at the end of this chapter for more information.

WHAT ARE THE PATHS TO BECOMING A NURSE?

- **Degree or diploma:** in England, you can get a diploma or a degree to get your basic qualification. In the other UK countries you must get a degree. A diploma course in England lasts 3 years. A degree course (in any of the UK countries) can be 3 or 4 years.
- **Nurse cadet:** in England, you can become a nurse cadet. Nurse cadets gain experience that leads to an NVQ 3 or to the Access to Nursing qualification. After getting those basics, cadets will go to university for their diploma course. This is a good route for people without formal qualifications who want to become nurses.
- **Access course:** you can also take the Access to Higher Education course (this is usually just called the 'Access course'). This equips adults who don't have formal qualifications like GCSEs or A levels, or who have been out of education for a while, with the skills and knowledge needed to enter higher education. The course for nursing is usually 1-year full time or 2 years part-time. You would take some useful courses like psychology, as well as learning how to study and take good notes.
- **Past experience:** sometimes, past experience can count for you. You can contact any local university and ask about accrediting prior and experiential learning (APEL) – a system that gives

you credit for your experience and learning. APEL may only count once you have been accepted onto the course.

- **Basic minimums:** if you already have the basic minimums (five GCSEs, or equivalent, at C or above, with English and a science), you can apply. You will find the list of contacts at the end of this chapter.

FUNDING

In England, funding is currently different for students on degree and diploma courses. Many student nurse groups have been actively lobbying the government to make the funding system more equitable, so with any luck by the time you are reading this there will be equal funding for both courses. At the moment, there are:

- means-tested bursaries for students on the degree course
- non-means-tested bursaries for diploma students.

Changes are currently taking place to child benefits and access to hardship funds and loans. You will need to contact the NHS Student Grants Unit for specific information on levels of support – it changes every year (details in the Contact section at the end of this chapter). In Wales, Scotland, and Northern Ireland there is a non-means-tested bursary for all nursing students.

The NHS pays for tuition and fees. You will need to buy your own books and pay for accommodation. You should have your uniforms provided (if you need them) through the university. Some travel costs may be reimbursed; you will need to find the current guideline by contacting either the Student Grants Unit or speaking to your university.

If you are an international student you will need further information about fees and bursaries as well as student visas. Contact the Nursing and Midwifery Admissions Service (NMAS) or the University and Colleges Admissions Service (UCAS) for up-to-date information (see Contacts section). Not all international students are eligible for free nurse training in the UK.

I can't afford to live on the bursary ...

Another way to become a nurse is to be seconded. This means that your employer pays for your education and pays you a salary while you are in university. You might or might not have to go back and work for that employer after you qualify.

Working as a health care assistant (HCA) in a hospital, or carer in a specialist area such as a learning disability or mental health setting can be an avenue into nursing. Speak to your human resources department about secondment opportunities.

Or you can take your nurse education in the military. Contact a recruiter for further information. Military nursing students have more demands placed on them but they also get a much higher level of financial support while they are students.

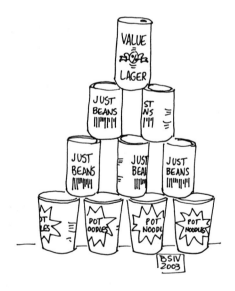

OK, you meet the entry requirements, have stocked up on baked beans and pot noodles, are ready to be skint for the next 3 or 4 years – now what?

CHOOSING YOUR UNIVERSITY

A number of factors will influence your choice of university:

- **Transport:** how will you get to class? Where will your placements be held and how will you get to them? Is there parking?
- **Accommodation:** where will you live when you are in uni, and how much will it cost?
- **The programme:** your course will be 3 or 4 years – is this the kind of place you want to spend the next 3 or 4 years?
- **The size:** nurse education programmes vary in size from very small to huge. You could have 40 people or 450 people in your class.
- **Resources:** how big is the library? Is there internet access? What is the tutor–student ratio?

When you contact NMAS or UCAS, they will send you a list of programmes. You can then find those in the area you live in, or where you want to live. Call those that interest you and ask them to send you information. You can also find out about them through:

- **Open days:** visiting a university, speaking to current students and finding out first hand what being a student there would be like is one of the best ways to know if you would be happy in the course there.
- **Quality Assurance Agency (QAA):** look-up the university on the QAA website (www.qaa.ac.uk). Nursing programmes are subject to audit – the QAA site will discuss the strengths and weakness of each course. You can then ask the uni what it is doing to improve areas the QAA site says are a problem!
- **Other nurses and nursing students:** talk to people. Go to online nurse discussion sites, ask people at work (if you work in healthcare), ask the practice nurse at your GP's surgery, ask people in the areas you think you might want to work in as a nurse. Be prepared to hear people advise you not to go into

nursing – some people are stressed and not very happy, and some people like to tease new students. Don't be put off by one bad report either – not everyone will have the same kinds of experiences.

- **A personal visit:** if you really like somewhere, call and ask for a tour and visit on your own. Visit the student union and ask about the course. Find where students are congregating and talk to them.

If all else fails and if, after you get in, you find it is just the wrong place for you, change to a different uni. After all, some trainees will find themselves moving house in the middle of their course. Changing to a different course can be complicated but it is usually possible.

I HAVE GOT ONTO A COURSE – NOW WHAT HAPPENS?

- **Your nursing course will be academically demanding:** make sure you have somewhere to keep your papers and books, and somewhere you can work in relative peace. You will accumulate quite a lot of paperwork, photocopies and handouts during your course – keeping it organized from the beginning will reduce the amount of time you spend wading through huge piles of paper looking for a handout from your first module when you are at the end of your second year!
- **You will need a diary:** from the beginning of your course until the day you qualify (and into your nursing career!) you will have a varied, often hectic schedule. A huge filofax tends to be a bit impractical (from personal experience) – a small academic (18-month) dairy is probably your best bet. As soon as you find out about classes, exams, assignment due dates, etc. write them down. Write down important contact details too, for friends, hospitals, wards, placement areas, tutors, etc. as you get them.

- **Don't go mad buying books:** you will need a decent nursing or medical dictionary, a drug calculations book and a study skills book. Oh, and *this book*. Of course! When the course starts, each module will tell you what is expected of you and will give a reading list. Don't buy a book until you know it will be useful – borrow it from the library first. Amazon (www. amazon.co.uk) and eBay (www.ebay.co.uk) sell second-hand nursing books at reduced rates.
- **Get to know the university ...**
  - There will usually be a bulletin board with messages about the course and a list of class sessions. Write down your class schedule as soon as you can but check back – arrangements often change.
  - Wander around and find all the different corridors and class-rooms. Get to know where the coffee shop is, where the loos are, where people relax. Nothing is worse than running late and not knowing where the classroom is.
  - Get to know everyone. It is amazing how often you will be glad that you made the effort to say 'Hello'.
  - Find the student union office and the learning resource centre/library.

If you will be living in student/university accommodation, have moved away from home for your nursing course, are an international/overseas student, are a recent school leaver or have any concerns or questions at all about life as a student, go to the student union office. They have some excellent publications (backed up by concerned and well informed staff!) to help you (see Appendix 1).

During the first few months you will be getting settled into your academic subjects and getting the mandatory training issues like lifting and handling out of the way. Many students say this is a difficult time – they want to just 'get into' nursing and get out on placements. It can be especially difficult if you have experience in healthcare. Be patient and enjoy the slow time – it soon will get so busy and hectic that the time will fly by. Plus, the information you get while waiting to 'get out there' is useful.

The common foundation programme

You will start on the common foundation programme (CFP). All students have the same basic first year then go into their specialized branches (these branches, as mentioned above, are adult, mental health nursing [see Appendix 2], learning disability [see Appendix 3] and children's nursing [see Appendix 4]). During your CFP you will be in lectures with nursing students from all the different branches. After CFP, you enter 'Branch'. Here, your education will be more specific to your chosen area of nursing and classes will probably be with those in the same branch. At the beginning of the course, you will have more academic time than placement time. By the end, you will be in placements most of the time. During the CFP you will probably take courses in:

- psychology and communication
- social influences on health
- basic nursing (skills and theories)
- how to study
- how to understand research
- anatomy and physiology (see Appendix 5 for list of normal lab values)
- community care
- social policy.

In Branch, courses may be similar but will be more specialized. For example, a children's nurse could take:

- acute care of the child
- health promotion for children and families
- child development.

During the CFP and Branch you will be expected to maintain a portfolio. This portfolio will be your proof of achievement. You will have the support of a personal tutor and other tutors in your programme. It will be up to you to maintain the portfolio and make certain that you have evidence of your achievements (more on portfolios in Chapter 10).

In practice, nurses in the placement areas will assess you. These nurses are your mentors and are responsible for helping you learn and gain clinical experience.

As you go on to further chapters in this book, there is a deeper discussion about academics and placements.

Just a note

Nurse education is physically, emotionally and financially stressful. Many students say that their relationships suffer during their courses and many also say that everything went wrong in their lives while they were getting their nursing qualification. It's an intense, hectic, demanding and stressful programme. Your friends on the course will help you - they know exactly what you are going through. Among my best friends are those I met on my nursing course. Make sure as well to set aside time for friends and family who aren't on the course. You being on the course will be tough on them, too.

When the course is over, things will stabilize. When it's over you will look back and wonder where the time went.

While you are on the course, remember: it will be terrible some days. It will have you stressed to the point of screaming. It will feel like it is never going to end. But there will also be days when you are walking on air and feel so happy you would like to dance on the ceiling. And then, before you know it, it will be over and you will be a nurse. You can do it!

REFERENCES

Henderson V 1966 *The nature of nursing*. Macmillan, New York
Royal College of Nursing 2003 *Defining nursing*. RCN, London

CONTACTS

The Nursing and Midwifery Council (NMC)
23 Portland Place, London, W1B 1PZ

Main switchboard: 020 7637 7181
Main fax: 020 7436 2924
Website: www.nmc-uk.org
E-mail: advice@nmc-uk.org

NHS Careers
Website: www.nhs.uk/careers
Provides general information about careers in nursing and midwifery, where nursing and midwifery courses are offered, how to apply for nursing and midwifery courses, funding, bursary information and other useful information.

Diploma courses (England)

The Nursing and Midwifery Admissions Service (NMAS)
Rosehill, New Barn Lane, Cheltenham, Gloucestershire, GL52 3LZ
Tel (application package): 01242 223707
Tel (general enquiries): 01242 544949
Fax: 01242 544962
Website: www.nmas.ac.uk

Degree courses

The University and Colleges Admissions Service (UCAS)
Barn Lane, Cheltenham, Gloucestershire, GL52 3LZ
Tel (application package): 01242 227788
Tel (general enquiries): 01242 222444
Fax: 01242 544961
Website: www.ucas.com

NHS information about nursing and nurse education

NHS Careers
PO Box 376, Bristol, BS99 3EY
Tel: 0845 60 60 655
Fax: 0117 921 9562
Website: www.nhs.uk/careers
E-mail: advice@nhscareers.nhs.uk

Department of Health

Department of Health
PO Box 777, London, SE1 6XH
For publications, e-mail: DOH@prologistics.co.uk

Financial and funding information in England

The NHS Student Grants Unit
22 Plymouth Road, Blackpool, FY3 7JS
Tel: 01253 655655
Fax: 01253 655660

Specific information about nursing and nurse education in Wales

NHS Professions Wales
2nd Floor, Golate House, 101 St Mary Street, Cardiff CF1 1DX
Tel: 02920 261400
Fax: 02920 261499
Website: www.wnb.org.uk
E-mail: info@wnb.org.uk

Financial and funding information in Wales

NHS Wales Students Awards Unit
2nd Floor Golate House, 101 St Mary Street, Cardiff, CF10 1DX

NHS Cymru Uned Dyfarniadau Myfyrwyr
2il Lawr Ty Golate, 101 Heol Eglwys Fair, Caerdydd, CF10 1DX

Tel: 02920 261495
Fax: 02920 261499

Specific information about nursing and nurse education in Scotland

NHS Education for Scotland
66 Rose Street, Edinburgh, EH2 2NN
Tel: 0131 225 4365
Website: www.nes.scot.nhs.uk
E-mail: careers@nes.scot.nhs.uk

Financial and funding information in Scotland

The Students Awards Agency for Scotland
3 Redheughs Rigg, South Gyle, Edinburgh, EH12 9HH
Tel: 0131 4768212

Specific information about nursing and nurse education in Northern Ireland

Queen's University Belfast
University Road, Belfast, BT7 1NN
Tel: 028 9024 5133
Fax: 028 9024 7895
Website: www.qub.ac.uk

Northern Ireland Practices and Educational Council (NIPEC)
Website: www.n-i.nhs.uk/nipec

Funding and financial information in Northern Ireland

The Department of Higher and Further Education Training and Employment
Student Support Branch, 4th Floor Adelaide House, 39-49 Adelaide Street, Belfast BT2 8FD
Tel: 028 9025 7777

What is the NMC?

2

> ❝ The NMC is here to protect the public ... ❞
> *Jonathan Asbridge, President of the NMC*

In this chapter

THE NMC

The Nursing and Midwifery Council (NMC) is an organization that ensures nurses, midwives and health visitors provide high standards of care to their patients and clients. Qualified nurses, midwives and health visitors are registered through the NMC, and the NMC has the right to suspend or remove practitioners from the register if it is proven that the practitioner is not safe, or does not behave in a professional manner.

The NMC also sets out guidelines and criteria for education and practice, gives advice to nurses, midwives and health visitors, and publishes numerous publications to support good practice. Among the NMC publications you will find most useful are:

- *Guidelines for Records and Record Keeping* (see Chapter 11, p. 192)

- *Guidelines for the Administration of Medicines* (see Chapter 8, p. 135)
- NMC *Code of Professional Conduct* (see p. 26)
- NMC *Guide for Students of Nursing and Midwifery* (see p. 34).

These publications are so important that they are included in this book. Please read them and refer back to them during your course. You can search the NMC website (www.nmc-uk.org) for information on many different subjects. Most NMC or UKCC publications are available on this website as a document file, or can be posted to you on request.

Before the NMC, the United Kingdom Central Council (UKCC) had these responsibilities. There was a national board in each of the four UK countries, which worked with the UKCC: these national boards have now been disbanded and, together with the UKCC, they became the NMC.

The one document with which most nurses are familiar is the NMC *Code of Professional Conduct*. This is like a rulebook for nursing, midwifery and health visiting – it tells you what is expected, what you should expect of others and highlights the criteria against which you will be measured should there ever be a complaint about your practice.

You will find the entire NMC *Code of Professional Conduct* on page 26–34. Please read it. For the most part, it is in plain English and is easy to understand.

When writing an assignment or a reflection, always try to find where the NMC Code fits in and cite it. It proves that you are aware of, and paying attention to, the guidelines set out for safe and competent practice. It will help you get good marks and become a responsible nurse. Also use the NMC Code when you are making decisions in your clinical area. The entire code is very long but don't be intimidated. The basic points are that, as a registered nurse, midwife or health visitor, you must:

- respect the patient or client as an individual
- obtain consent before you give any treatment or care

- cooperate with others in the team
- protect confidential information
- maintain your professional knowledge and competence
- be trustworthy
- act to identify and minimize the risk to patients and clients.

The NMC *Guide for Students of Nursing and Midwifery* (see pp 34–37) is very easy to read and really gives you important information and support. It explains how the Code of Conduct applies to you, and how you are expected to act as a student nurse. I have included these two documents in this chapter to highlight how important they are if you are to become a safe and competent practitioner. I cannot overemphasize how much these documents can help you in your course. The main points of the NMC *Guide for Students of Nursing and Midwifery* are that:

- You must always work under the supervision of a qualified nurse or midwife, as you are not accountable under the NMC *Code of Professional Conduct*. You are, however, responsible for working within the limitations of your role as a student.
- You must always identify yourself as a student nurse. You must always let patients and their families know that you are a student, and you must identify yourself as a student on the telephone. Patients have a right to say 'No' to having a student care for them.
- You have an obligation to maintain patient confidentiality.
- You must never do *anything* that is outside your role as a student.

When you finish your course (and, yes – there is light at the end of the nursing education tunnel!) you will register with the NMC. The way it currently works is:

1. You successfully finish your course (thinking '… and am I glad I had the *Student Nurse Handbook* …').

2. Your uni sends the NMC a list of graduates and affirms that you, as individuals, are of 'good character'. This declaration is an essential part of your process to join the register (don't worry: if there are any concerns, you will know about them before it gets to this point) – make absolutely certain that your uni spells your name properly and sends the NMC your current address.

3. The NMC sends your registering information, asks you to confirm your name and address, and tells you where to send the registration fee. Remember: if someone else is paying for your fees for you (which is likely because you will be pretty skint at this point in your student career), make sure your name, address and NMC personal identification number (PIN) is on the cheque.

4. You wait. Registration doesn't take as long as it used to but the wait is still nerve wracking. You have waited all this time to be a real nurse and you ache to wear the blue uniform ... and get the nurse's pay! Although you will probably be paid as an HCA while you are waiting for your PIN to be added to the register, most employers pay you the higher rate retrospectively once it comes through. Remember: you cannot call yourself a nurse until your PIN is registered.

5. When your PIN comes through, call your employer and let them know. They have a special contact at the NMC to confirm your registration.

Something to think about: you will now, if you are normal, go absolutely money mad. Clothes, a car – all those things that have been waiting while you were a student – are suddenly within your reach. It will be very easy to get credit too. The joy of finishing your course, getting a real job and finally being a nurse can mute your common sense a bit so don't get ahead of yourself and spend all your money!

When your PIN comes through, you are a card-carrying nurse. You are now accountable under the *Code of Professional Conduct* and, in the not-too-distant future, a student nurse will be working with you, looking up to you, and wondering 'Will I ever be able to do what he (or she) does?' just like you did with your mentor. Please, don't get qualified-nurse-amnesia: never forget what it was like to be a student. You know how frustrating and stressful it is; you know what a difference a good and interested mentor can make. If you had bad mentors, the best way to make up for it is always to be a good one.

REFERENCES

Nursing and Midwifery Council 2002 Code of professional conduct. NMC, London
Nursing and Midwifery Council 2002 Guide for students of nursing and midwifery. NMC, London

CONTACTS

NMC
23 Portland Place, London, W1B 1PZ

Telephone enquiries:

- Main switchboard: 020 7637 7181
- Registrations: 020 7333 9333
- Overseas applications: 020 7333 6600
- Employer Confirmations: 020 7631 3200
- Fitness to Practise: 020 7333 6564
- Professional advice: 020 7333 6550
- Press enquiries: 020 7333 6557/6558

Website: www.nmc-uk.org

Appendix 2.1: NMC *Code of Professional Conduct*

As a registered nurse, midwife or health visitor, you are personally accountable for your practice. In caring for patients and clients, you must:

- respect the patient or client as an individual
- obtain consent before you give any treatment or care
- protect confidential information
- cooperate with others in the team
- maintain your professional knowledge and competence
- be trustworthy
- act to identify and minimize risk to patients and clients.

These are the shared values of all the United Kingdom health care regulatory bodies.

1   Introduction

1.1   The purpose of the *Code of Professional Conduct* is to:

- inform the professions of the standard of professional conduct required of them in the exercise of their professional accountability and practice
- inform the public, other professions and employers of the standard of professional conduct that they can expect of a registered practitioner.

1.2   As a registered nurse, midwife or health visitor, you must:

- protect and support the health of individual patients and clients
- protect and support the health of the wider community
- act in such a way that justifies the trust and confidence the public have in you
- uphold and enhance the good reputation of the professions.

1.3   You are personally accountable for your practice. This means that you are answerable for your actions and omissions, regardless of advice or directions from another professional.

1.4   You have a duty of care to your patients and clients, who are entitled to receive safe and competent care.

1.5   You must adhere to the laws of the country in which you are practising.

2 As a registered nurse, midwife or health visitor, you must respect the patient or client as an individual

2.1 You must recognize and respect the role of patients and clients as partners in their care and the contribution they can make to it. This involves identifying their preferences regarding care and respecting these within the limits of professional practice, existing legislation, resources and the goals of the therapeutic relationship.

2.2 You are personally accountable for ensuring that you promote and protect the interests and dignity of patients and clients, irrespective of gender, age, race, ability, sexuality, economic status, lifestyle, culture and religious or political beliefs.

2.3 You must, at all times, maintain appropriate professional boundaries in the relationships you have with patients and clients. You must ensure that all aspects of the relationship focus exclusively upon the needs of the patient or client.

2.4 You must promote the interests of patients and clients. This includes helping individuals and groups gain access to health and social care, information and support relevant to their needs.

2.5 You must report to a relevant person or authority, at the earliest possible time, any conscientious objection that may be relevant to your professional practice. You must continue to provide care to the best of your ability until alternative arrangements are implemented.

3 As a registered nurse, midwife or health visitor, you must obtain consent before you give any treatment or care

3.1 All patients and clients have a right to receive information about their condition. You must be sensitive to their needs and respect the wishes of those who refuse or are unable to receive information about their condition. Information should be accurate, truthful and presented in such a way as to make it easily understood. You may need to seek legal or professional advice, or guidance from your employer, in relation to the giving or withholding of consent.

3.2   You must respect patients' and clients' autonomy – their right to decide whether or not to undergo any health care intervention – even where a refusal may result in harm or death to themselves or a foetus, unless a court of law orders to the contrary. This right is protected in law, although in circumstances where the health of the foetus would be severely compromised by any refusal to give consent, it would be appropriate to discuss this matter fully within the team, and possibly to seek external advice and guidance (see clause 4).

3.3   When obtaining valid consent, you must be sure that it is:
- given by a legally competent person
- given voluntarily
- informed.

3.4   You should presume that every patient and client is legally competent unless otherwise assessed by a suitably qualified practitioner. A patient or client who is legally competent can understand and retain treatment information and can use it to make an informed choice.

3.5   Those who are legally competent may give consent in writing, orally or by cooperation. They may also refuse consent. You must ensure that all your discussions and associated decisions relating to obtaining consent are documented in the patient's or client's health care records.

3.6   When patients or clients are no longer legally competent and thus have lost the capacity to consent to or refuse treatment and care, you should try to find out whether they have previously indicated preferences in an advance statement. You must respect any refusal of treatment or care given when they were legally competent, provided that the decision is clearly applicable to the present circumstances and that there is no reason to believe that they have changed their minds. When such a statement is not available, the patients' or clients' wishes, if known, should be taken into account. If these wishes are not known, the criteria for treatment must be that it is in their best interests.

3.7   The principles of obtaining consent apply equally to those people who have a mental illness. Whilst you should be involved in their assessment, it will also be necessary to involve relevant people close to them; this may include a psychiatrist. When patients and clients are detained under statutory powers (mental health acts), you must ensure that you know the circumstances and safeguards needed for providing treatment and care without consent.

3.8   In emergencies where treatment is necessary to preserve life, you may provide care without patients' or clients' consent, if they are unable to give it, provided you can demonstrate that you are acting in their best interests.

3.9   No-one has the right to give consent on behalf of another competent adult. In relation to obtaining consent for a child, the involvement of those with parental responsibility in the consent procedure is usually necessary, but will depend on the age and understanding of the child. If the child is under the age of 16 in England and Wales, 12 in Scotland and 17 in Northern Ireland, you must be aware of legislation and local protocols relating to consent.

3.10 Usually the individual performing a procedure should be the person to obtain the patient's or client's consent. In certain circumstances, you may seek consent on behalf of colleagues if you have been specially trained for that specific area of practice.

3.11 You must ensure that the use of complementary or alternative therapies is safe and in the interests of patients and clients. This must be discussed with the team as part of the therapeutic process and the patient or client must consent to their use.

4   As a registered nurse, midwife or health visitor, you must cooperate with others in the team

4.1   The team includes the patient or client, the patient's or client's family, informal carers and health and social care professionals in the National Health Service, independent and voluntary sectors.

4.2   You are expected to work co-operatively within teams and to respect the skills, expertise and contributions of your colleagues. You must treat them fairly and without discrimination.

4.3   You must communicate effectively and share your knowledge, skill and expertise with other members of the team as required for the benefit of patients and clients.

4.4   Health care records are a tool of communication within the team. You must ensure that the health care record for the patient or client is an accurate account of treatment, care planning and delivery. It should be consecutive, written with the involvement of the patient or client wherever practicable and completed as soon as possible after an event has occurred. It should provide clear evidence of the care planned, the decisions made, the care delivered and the information shared.

4.5   When working as a member of a team, you remain accountable for your professional conduct, any care you provide and any omission on your part.

4.6   You may be expected to delegate care delivery to others who are not registered nurses or midwives. Such delegation must not compromise existing care but must be directed to meeting the needs and serving the interests of patients and clients. You remain accountable for the appropriateness of the delegation, for ensuring that the person who does the work is able to do it and that adequate supervision or support is provided.

4.7   You have a duty to co-operate with internal and external investigations.

5   As a registered nurse, midwife or health visitor, you must protect confidential information

5.1   You must treat information about patients and clients as confidential and use it only for the purposes for which it was given. As it is impractical to obtain consent every time you need to share information with others, you should ensure that patients and clients understand that some information may be made available to other members of the team involved in the delivery of care. You must guard against breaches of confidentiality by protecting information from improper disclosure at all times.

5.2   You should seek patients' and clients' wishes regarding the sharing of information with their family and others. When a patient or client is considered incapable of giving permission, you should consult relevant colleagues.

5.3   If you are required to disclose information outside the team that will have personal consequences for patients or clients, you must obtain their consent. If the patient or client withholds consent, or if consent cannot be obtained for whatever reason, disclosures may be made only where:

- they can be justified in the public interest (usually where disclosure is essential to protect the patient or client or someone else from the risk of significant harm)
- they are required by law or by order of a court.

5.4   Where there is an issue of child protection, you must act at all times in accordance with national and local policies.

6   As a registered nurse, midwife or health visitor, you must maintain your professional knowledge and competence

6.1   You must keep your knowledge and skills up-to-date throughout your working life. In particular, you should take part regularly in learning activities that develop your competence and performance.

6.2   To practise competently, you must possess the knowledge, skills and abilities required for lawful, safe and effective practice without direct supervision. You must acknowledge the limits of your professional competence and only undertake practice and accept responsibilities for those activities in which you are competent.

6.3   If an aspect of practice is beyond your level of competence or outside your area of registration, you must obtain help and supervision from a competent practitioner until you and your employer consider that you have acquired the requisite knowledge and skill.

6.4   You have a duty to facilitate students of nursing, midwifery and health visiting and others to develop their competence.

6.5   You have a responsibility to deliver care based on current evidence, best practice and, where applicable, validated research when it is available.

7   As a registered nurse, midwife or health visitor, you must be trustworthy

7.1   You must behave in a way that upholds the reputation of the professions. Behaviour that compromises this reputation may call your registration into question even if it is not directly connected to your professional practice.

7.2   You must ensure that your registration status is not used in the promotion of commercial products or services, declare any financial or other interests in relevant organizations providing such goods or services and ensure that your professional judgement is not influenced by any commercial considerations.

7.3   When providing advice regarding any product or service relating to your professional role or area of practice, you must be aware of the risk that, on account of your professional title or qualification, you could be perceived by the patient or client as endorsing the product. You should fully explain the advantages and disadvantages of alternative products so that the patient or client can make an informed choice. Where you recommend a specific product, you must ensure that your advice is based on evidence and is not for your own commercial gain.

7.4   You must refuse any gift, favour or hospitality that might be interpreted, now or in the future, as an attempt to obtain preferential consideration.

7.5   You must neither ask for nor accept loans from patients, clients or their relatives and friends.

8   As a registered nurse, midwife or health visitor, you must act to identify and minimize the risk to patients and clients

8.1   You must work with other members of the team to promote health care environments that are conducive to safe, therapeutic and ethical practice.

8.2   You must act quickly to protect patients and clients from risk if you have good reason to believe that you or a colleague, from your own or another profession, may not be fit to practise for reasons of conduct, health or competence. You should be aware of the terms of legislation that offer protection for people who raise concerns about health and safety issues.

8.3   Where you cannot remedy circumstances in the environment of care that could jeopardize standards of practice, you must report them to a senior person with sufficient authority to manage them and also, in the case of midwifery, to the supervisor of midwives. This must be supported by a written record.

8.4   When working as a manager, you have a duty toward patients and clients, colleagues, the wider community and the organization in which you and your colleagues work. When facing professional dilemmas, your first consideration in all activities must be the interests and safety of patients and clients.

8.5 In an emergency, in or outside the work setting, you have a professional duty to provide care. The care provided would be judged against what could reasonably be expected from someone with your knowledge, skills and abilities when placed in those particular circumstances.

Glossary

Accountable: Responsible for something or to someone.
Care: To provide help or comfort.
Competent: Possessing the skills and abilities required for lawful, safe and effective professional practice without direct supervision.
Patient and client: Any individual or group using a health service.
Reasonable: The case of Bolam *v* Friern Hospital Management Committee (1957) produced the following definition of what is reasonable: 'The test is the standard of the ordinary skilled man exercising and professing to have that special skill. A man need not possess the highest expert skill at the risk of being found negligent ... it is sufficient if he exercises the skill of an ordinary man exercising that particular art.' This definition is supported and clarified by the case of Bolitho *v* City and Hackney Health Authority (1993).

Further information

This *Code of Professional Conduct* is available on the Nursing and Midwifery Council's website at www.nmc-uk.org. Printed copies can be obtained by writing to the Publications Department, Nursing and Midwifery Council, 23 Portland Place, London W1B 1PZ, by fax on 020 7436 2924 or by e-mail at publications@nmc-uk.org.

A wide range of NMC standards and guidance publications expand upon and develop many of the professional issues and themes identified in the *Code of Professional Conduct*. All are available on the NMC's website. A list of current NMC publications is available either on the website or on request from the Publications Department as above.

Enquiries about the issues addressed in the *Code of Professional Conduct* should be directed in the first instance to the NMC's professional advice service at the address above, by e-mail at advice@nmc-uk.org, by telephone on 020 7333 6541/6550/6553 or by fax on 020 7333 6538.

The Nursing and Midwifery Council will keep this *Code of Professional Conduct* under review and any comments, suggestions or requests for further clarification are welcome, both from practitioners and members of the public. These should be addressed to the Director of Policy and Standards, NMC, 23 Portland Place, London W1B 1PZ.

Summary

As a registered nurse, midwife or health visitor, you must:

- respect the patient or client as an individual
- obtain consent before you give any treatment or care
- cooperate with others in the team
- protect confidential information
- maintain your professional knowledge and competence
- be trustworthy
- act to identify and minimize the risk to patients and clients.

Reproduced with permission of the NMC.

Appendix 2.2: NMC *Guide for Students of Nursing and Midwifery*

As a pre-registration student of nursing or midwifery, you will already have started to think about your future career as a registered nurse or midwife. Once you have successfully completed your programme of education, you will need to register with the Nursing and Midwifery Council (NMC) before you can practise as a nurse or midwife. This leaflet sets out some basic information about the NMC and some guidance for the clinical experience you will undertake during your studies. It is based upon extensive consultation with individual pre-registration students of nursing and midwifery, organizations representing students and lecturers in higher education. The leaflet should be read in conjunction with advice provided by your higher education institution.

What does the NMC do?

The NMC is the regulatory body for nursing and midwifery. Our purpose is to establish and improve standards of nursing and midwifery care in order to protect the public. These standards are set out in the *Code of Professional Conduct*, which the NMC will send to you when you first register. We urge you to get hold of a copy now. You should be able to obtain it through your university; if not, please write to our Publications Department. You may not be aware that the standards set by the NMC already apply to you.

The level of entry to the programme of education that you are undertaking and the content, type and length of your programme are all part of these standards. Our other key tasks are to:

- maintain a register of qualified nurses and midwives
- set standards for nursing and midwifery education, practice and conduct

- provide advice for nurses and midwives on professional standards
- consider allegations of misconduct or unfitness to practise due to ill health.

Registration and professional accountability

When you successfully complete your course, your higher education institution will notify the NMC that you have met the required standards and that you are eligible for entry on the register. Your course director will also complete a declaration of good character form on your behalf. When we have received this information and you have paid your registration fee, your name will be entered on the NMC register and you will be eligible to practise as a registered practitioner.

Registration is not simply an administrative process. The NMC's register is an instrument of public protection and anyone can check the registered status of a nurse or midwife. Registering with the NMC demonstrates that you have met the standards expected of registered nurses and midwives. It also demonstrates that you are professionally accountable at all times for your acts and omissions.

Professional accountability involves weighing up the interests of patients, using your professional judgement and skills to make a decision and enabling you to account for the decision you make. On rare occasions, nurses and midwives fall short of the professional standards expected of them. The NMC investigates in the public interest any complaints made about the professional conduct or fitness to practise of registered nurses and midwives.

Throughout your career, you will need to keep up to date with developments in your area of practice. Your continuing professional development is an integral part of your professional accountability. In order to continue to practise, you will need to meet the NMC's standards for post-registration education and practice (PREP).

Detailed information about PREP is available in *The PREP Handbook*, which you can obtain free of charge by writing to the Publications Department. You will also need to complete a notification of practice form and pay your periodic registration fee when you renew your registration every three years. Practising midwives also need to complete a notification of intention to practise form annually.

Guidance on clinical experience for students

During your studentship, you will come into close contact with patients. This may be through observing care being given, through helping in providing care and, later, through full participation in providing care. At all times, you should work only within your level of understanding and competence and always under the direct supervision of a registered nurse or midwife. The section below provides some guidance on working with patients during your studies. The principles underpinning this guidance reflect the standards that will be expected of you when you become a registered practitioner.

Your accountability

As a pre-registration student, you are *never* professionally accountable in the way that you will be after you come to register with the NMC. This means that you cannot be called to account for your actions and omissions by the NMC. So far as the NMC is concerned, it is the registered practitioners with whom you are working who are professionally responsible for the consequences of your actions and omissions. This is why you must always work under the direct supervision of a registered nurse or midwife. This does not mean, however, that you can never be called to account by your university or by the law for the consequences of your actions or omissions as a pre-registration student.

The wishes of patients

You must respect the wishes of patients at all times. They have the right to refuse to allow you, as a student, to participate in caring for them and you should make this right clear to them when they are first given information about the care they will receive from you. You should leave if they ask you to do so. Their rights as patients supersede at all times your rights to knowledge and experience.

Identifying yourself

Introduce yourself accurately at all times when speaking to patients either directly or by telephone. In doing so, you should make it quite clear that you are a pre-registration student and not a registered practitioner. In fact, it is a criminal offence to represent yourself falsely and deliberately as a registered nurse or midwife.

Accepting appropriate responsibility

You will find yourself at times in a position where you may not be directly accompanied by your mentor, supervisor or another registered colleague. You will also experience emergencies. As your skills, experience and confidence develop, you will become increasingly able to deal with these situations. However, as a student, do not participate in any procedure for which you have not been fully prepared or in which you are not adequately supervised. If such a situation arises, discuss the matter as quickly as possible with your supervisor.

Patient confidentiality

Patients have the right to know that any private and personal information that is given in confidence will be used only for the purposes for which it was originally provided and that it will not be used for any other reason. If you want to refer in a written assignment to some real-life situation in which you have been involved, do not provide any information that could identify a particular patient. Obtain access to patient records only when absolutely necessary for the care being provided.

Use of these records must be closely supervised by a registered practitioner and you must follow the local policy on the handling and storage of records. Any written entry you make in a patient's records must be counter-signed by a registered practitioner. You can find more advice about confidentiality in the NMC's *Code of Professional Conduct*. You should also refer to our *Guidelines for Records and Record Keeping*.

Handling complaints

Be aware of the local procedures for dealing with complaints by patients, or their families, about the treatment or care they are receiving. If patients indicate to you that they are unhappy about their treatment or care, you should report the matter immediately to the person who is supervising your clinical experience or to another appropriate person.

Published by the former United Kingdom Central Council for Nursing, Midwifery and Health Visiting in July 1998. Reprinted by the Nursing and Midwifery Council in April 2002.

We hope that you will find these notes helpful during your studentship and in understanding the important responsibilities you will undertake as a registered nurse or midwife. If you need to discuss any of these issues with us, please contact our professional advice service on 020 7333 6541/6550/6553, by e-mail at advice@nmc-uk.org or by fax on 020 7333 6538. If you would like to find out more about the work of the NMC, please write to our Publications Department for a list of current publications. The NMC's website at www.nmc-uk.org includes copies of all NMC publications, position statements issued by our professional advice service and further useful information and contacts for students of nursing and midwifery. We wish you success in your programme of preparation for registration and in your future career.

Reproduced with permission of the NMC.

Nursing Models

3

❛ It took me a while to get my head around all the different models, but now that I have been in a number of placements I am starting to understand how useful they are ... They are a road map to delivering good care. ❜

Second-year student nurse

In this chapter

During your course, you will probably have at least one module that looks at nursing models and frameworks, and at the influence nursing models have on the delivery of care. This doesn't mean that this is the only place you will discuss them: nursing models and frameworks are in the background of most of the things you will do as a nurse, so of course they are in the background of most things you will do as a student! So, why do you need to know them?

- you will have modules about them
- you will need to use them for material in assessments in different modules
- you will use them on your placements

- you will take parts of them and use them to do your work as a nurse
- it makes you look brilliant when you know about them!

Here are some terms for you:

- nursing
- nursing process
- holism
- holistic care
- philosophy
- nursing theory
- framework
- model/nursing model.

You will need to use these terms throughout your course and into your career.

NURSING

There is no way to define nursing succinctly, because each individual nurse comes into nursing with his or her own beliefs, skills and interests. There was more about the meaning of nursing in Chapter 1 but it's important to think about it again here because all the nursing models and theories stem from beliefs about the meaning of nursing. Viriginia Henderson (1966) gave us one of the most common and universal descriptions of nursing:

> ❝ The unique function of the nurse is to assist the individual, sick or well, in the performance of those activities contributing to health or its recovery (or to peaceful death) that he would perform unaided if he had the necessary strength, will, or knowledge. And to do this in such a way as to help him gain independence as rapidly as possible. ❞

Basically, Henderson says that nurses do for patients what they would do for themselves if they were able. In her discussion about nursing, Henderson identifies the different ways in which nurses assist patients, but emphasizes that the ultimate goal of nursing care is to help the individual to gain independence. Her definition tells us that nurses need to help patients find strength, to provide education to improve patients' knowledge, and help the patients make the best decisions about their health and their care.

NURSING PROCESS

In the 1960s, when Virginia Henderson's definition of nursing was first published, nursing was beginning a period of dramatic change. It was growing out of being a service profession that existed only to do hygiene care and work as directed by doctors and was becoming recognized as a profession in its own right. Nursing theorists were beginning really to look at the way nurses were thinking. One result of this was the development of the 'nursing process', an explanation of a way of making decisions and thinking about how to deliver care.

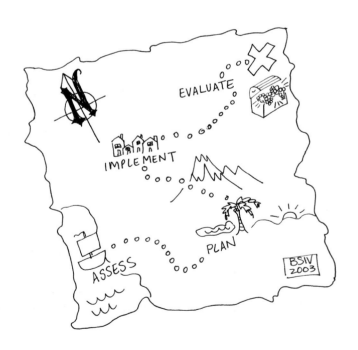

You can use the nursing process in a number of ways: care planning, writing nurse's notes or simply just making sure that you are using good judgement when making decisions in practice are all examples of the nursing process. There is nothing magical about it: it is simply an organized way of thinking.

There are four steps in a nursing process:

1. **Assess:** make a full assessment of the situation.
2. **Plan:** what do you want to accomplish? What goals do you have for this patient/situation?
3. **Implement:** how will you accomplish the goals?
4. **Evaluate:** how did your implementation work towards achieving the goals you set? Do you need a new plan or new method of implementation?

The nursing process isn't an entity by itself – it is a process through which you make decisions, record information, and so on. It is useful in more than just nursing as well: try it next time you pack for holiday!

HOLISM

The NMC *Code of Professional Conduct* (NMC 2002) tells you that you must respect the client as an individual. This means that you must look at all the different elements that make up your patient: the body, the mind and the spiritual self. This is the basis of holism.

HOLISTIC CARE

Holism and holistic care look at the patient as a whole person, with unique and individual needs and circumstances. Holism drives the nurse to see more than just the reason patients are in care: it encourages them to look at the way patients feel, what is important to them and their families, the details of their living situation, what they believe, etc.

When discussing holism you come across buzz words such as 'spiritual', 'emotional', 'physiological', 'psychological' and 'cultural'. Try not to worry about what these mean, just try to remember that there is more to your patient than being a patient. If you see your patients in '3-D', you will give the care that best meets all their needs in a respectful and dignified way. This means remembering *never* to stereotype a patient: there is no such thing as an 'average Asian patient'; people who are Muslim will not always follow a halal diet; not all Afro-Caribbean people eat chicken and rice and not every Asian person wants a vegetarian curry for tea. Don't assume, based on someone's name or appearance, that you know what his or her needs are. How would you feel if someone thought of you as being 'average British' and fed you nothing but fish and chips? Just because someone is from a particular culture doesn't mean they do all the things that you might believe are done in that culture.

Making sure that you approach care in a holistic way can be difficult. That's why we use nursing models and frameworks to guide us. Nursing models, theories and frameworks are all related. Here's how they develop: an individual looks at nursing and identifies his or her philosophy. Next, he or she starts to think about nursing, about nursing care, and about the best way to meet the patient's needs. This develops into a theory. The theory then develops into a model. From the model, the individual can develop a framework – a way for the model to be applied to nursing. At some level, we are all nursing theorists, because each of us develops our own beliefs, ideas and approaches to care.

The way you approach care is founded in your philosophy. Each of us has our own philosophy, even if we don't think about it actively. It can be important for your development and growth as a nurse to think about and reflect on your beliefs about nursing, the values nurses hold and the way nurses approach care.

PHILOSOPHY

A nursing philosophy is the principle a nurse, placement area or organization uses to guide the approach they have to patients, care and care delivery. Look for the philosophy in any area you are placed in and ask yourself:

- If I were a patient, or member of staff, could I find it?
- If I were a patient, would I feel this applies to me/my care?
- Does it make sense?
- Is it too long to read? Is it too short to mean anything?
- Is it too full of buzz words to have real meaning?
- Would a staff member be able to have confidence in this?
- Would staff members say this reflects their beliefs?
- Does it make sense? Is it too idealist or too vague?
- How was it developed? Did current staff have input?
- Is it ever reviewed or updated?
- Does it reflect holism?
- Does it conflict with the *Code of Professional Conduct* in any way?

A philosophy isn't something that can simply be handed to people, it has to be something they believe in. You can learn a surprising amount about the area by looking at the philosophy: it will tell you not just what the area wants to say it believes, but about management, staff involvement and morale.

Individuals also have their own philosophy. Each of us does – we just don't often put it into words. I had a philosophy in mind when I started this book: I wanted it to be clear, direct, friendly and useful. I have my own philosophy of nursing as well. So do you. In Chapter 6, I challenge you to write it down – if you've already done that, then bravo! If not, think about it now … write down 'I believe that nursing is …' and 'I believe that as a nurse I …' This is important. You will have a clearer vision of what you are trying to achieve if you put it into words. It will help you to centre and focus yourself when you get stressed and discouraged. It will help you make better decisions if you know why you are in practice.

So, you know what you believe (your philosophy) and you know you want to address patients and their needs in a way that considers all the different aspects of their lives. You need a framework to help you, to make sure that you approach your care in an organized way and so that nothing gets left out.

NURSING THEORY

Nursing theory is a belief or understanding about the way things are done, or should be done, in nursing. A nursing theory is an organized way of looking at nursing, nursing care and the knowledge contained in nursing. Through nursing theories, nursing practice is explored, gaps in knowledge are investigated and research is generated. This is based on a philosophy about nursing and values held by the theorist that is believed to be important. The theory is then developed, through research, investigation, audit and observation. The theory can then develop into a model – an organized approach to care based on the theory. Nursing theories are the foundation of knowledge that supports nursing practice.

FRAMEWORK

A nursing framework is the way a nurse organizes the care delivered to the patient. It is based on a nursing model (or a combination of models). There are different kinds of frameworks: some are meant to be on paper, some are meant to be in your head (conceptual frameworks) and some are meant to be both. An example of a paper framework is an assessment sheet that you fill in. The nursing process is an example of a framework that is in your head. Don't rely on the paper frameworks alone. It's up to you as a nurse to have a clear vision for the way you approach your care. Frameworks are built as an expression of the different models.

MODELS

A model is an example or a pattern. A nursing model is based on a philosophy that someone had about care and nursing. This developed into a theoretical approach to care and, from there, became an example and explanation of a way to apply that theory. There are many different nursing models (and theories) and many different nursing theorists. They all have some things in common, and many of them are quite similar.

You will find that different models use different perspectives to look at patients and their care. Some models (like those developed by Roper, Logan and Tierney) look specifically at meeting the patient's needs. Other models (like Watson's) look at the nurse's interaction with the patient. Still other models will focus on the patient's environment and their adaptation within it. When looking at nursing models, try to identify the approach the theorist is taking. This will help you understand what it is the model expects you to do to care for the patient. Basing an approach to care on more than one model is being 'eclectic'.

Roper (the activities of living model)

The Roper model – developed by Roper, Logan and Tierney (2002) – has five sections, of which only one (the activities of living) tends to be used in the placement area. This asks the nurse to assess the patient based on life skills and needs such as eating and dressing, maintaining body temperature and being able to walk. The model was designed to look at how dependent someone is on assistance from others. One key feature many people ignore in the Roper model is that any assessment of activities of living (AL) needs to look holistically at the patient. Roper specifies five key aspects that must be considered when assessing ALs: biological, psychological, sociocultural, environmental and politicoeconomic. This model is based on the Henderson theory of nursing.

King

The focus of King's model is '… on individuals whose interactions in groups within social systems influence behaviour within the systems' (King 1989). The experiences people have in their environment, and the perceptions people have about the world around them, influence their behaviour and, as a result, their health and wellness.

King's model looks at personal, interpersonal and social interactions. In this model, the nurse works together with the client to determine and work towards goals and solutions (goal attaintment).

Orem (the self-care deficit model)

In this model, the nurse must identify what patients can – and can't – do for themselves and then identify how best to help patients overcome the deficit between the two. The nurse must also identify areas where patients need education, information, support or advice to become more independent and to address any health or lifestyle problems. This is a very popular model in the United States.

Peplau (the interpersonal relations model)

Peplau emphasizes the development of a trusting therapeutic relationship between nurse and patient. The nurse and patient progress through phases as they proceed with the interpersonal process of developing this relationship. There is an emphasis on developing patients' knowledge and ability to cope, and to help them learn the skills and knowledge they need to attain and maintain health. The role of the nurse is to identify behaviour that interferes with health, to develop a therapeutic relationship and, through this relationship, to help patients overcome that behaviour. There is a focus on therapeutic communication. The model states that nursing is a 'significant, therapeutic interpersonal process'.

Leininger (the transcultural nursing model)

The Leininger model emphasizes care '… focused upon differences and similarities among cultures with respect to human care, health, and illness based upon the people's cultural values, beliefs, and practices, and to use this knowledge to provide cultural specific or culturally congruent nursing care to people' (Leininger 1978).

Levine (Levine's conservation model)

The nurse assesses the patient's adaptation – both personally and socially – and then supports that patient in making the necessary changes to attain and maintain 'wholeness'. The nurse helps the patient conserve energy by helping the patient to adapt appropriately to the environment.

Neuman

In Neuman's model, the nurse is the leader of the healthcare team because the nurse's broad scope encompasses all the patient's needs. The goal is to help individuals achieve, and maintain, the optimum level of health possible. It encourages the nurse to identify and to help the individual identify stressors in the environment that can be controlled, helping the individual to return to a more stable, healthy state. This return to a healthy state is called 'reconstitution'. This is related to Roger's theory of energy fields.

Rogers (unitary health care model)

The Rogers model is a complicated theory that looks at neither health nor illness, but instead focuses on patterns of energy: it looks at energy fields as the basic units of living (and non-living) things. The interaction between energy fields affects the patterns of the fields. I personally find this an interesting but chaotic and difficult model to follow.

Roy (Roy's adaptive model)

In this model, the nurse is asked to see patients relative to their environment, and to assist them in adapting, in a positive way, to the circumstances in which they find themselves. Roy sees patients as people with biological, psychological and social aspects. The patients must adapt to their environment: they do this through changes in their body, in their function, in the way they see themselves and in the level of dependence they have on other people. To protect themselves, they use different coping skills. It is up to the nurse to help patients develop good coping skills, and to help them identify and resolve any negative coping skills.

Watson (theory of caring)

Watson outlines a number of elements in her model but they all boil down to: be genuinely caring, give hope, have faith and develop therapeutic relationships, founded in non-judgemental communication, that sensitively nurture patients and their families.

There are many other nursing theorists. This chapter isn't intended to teach you everything you will ever need to know about nursing models and theories but rather to give you a head start at identifying some of the basic theories and key themes you will encounter in your course. If you want to know more, there is a lot of information on the internet: just type the name of the model or the nursing theorist who developed it into a search engine.

One note here: nursing theory and models are living things. They are used, adapted, modified and reworked. Each one contributes to the body of knowledge and practice of nursing, and as each one follows another, incorporates elements that have gone before. Nothing in nursing theory is a 'stand alone' concept. What that should tell you about nursing itself is that there is room for interpretation. This is exactly the reason I am encouraging you to develop your own philosophy about nursing. You don't have to choose one model to follow: find what works for you.

Summary

- Every nurse has his or her own philosophy of nursing.
- Holism and holistic care look at each individual as an individual with individual needs, concerns and qualities.

- There are many different nursing models: most nurses use an eclectic combination of models and frameworks in their work.

- There is no 'right' or 'wrong' model or theory: each has points that a nurse could find useful, but some are more useful than others.

- Philosophies for clinical areas should reflect the current beliefs and values of the people working there.

REFERENCES

Heather A, Roy C 1999 The Roy adaptation model, 2nd edn. Prentice Hall, New Jersey

Henderson V 1966 The nature of nursing. Macmillan, New York

King I M 1989 King's general systems framework and theory. In: Riehl-Sisca J P (ed) Conceptual models for nursing practice, 3rd edn. Appleton & Lange, Norwalk, CT

Kozier B, Erb G, Blais K et al 1998 Fundamentals of nursing: concepts, process, and practice, 5th edn. Addison Wesley Longman, Menlo Park, CA

Leininger M (ed) 1978 Transcultural nursing. Wiley, New York

Neuman B, Fawcett J (eds) 2002 The Neuman systems model, 4th edn. Prentice Hall, Upper Saddle River, NJ

Nursing and Midwifery Council 2002 Code of professional conduct. NMC, London

Peplau H E 1991 Interpersonal relations in nursing: a conceptual framework of reference for psychodynamic nursing. Springer Publishing, New York

Riehl-Sisca J (ed) 1989 Conceptual models for nursing practice, 3rd edn. Appleton & Lange, Norwalk, CT

Rogers M 1983 Science of unitary human beings: A paradigm for nursing. In: Clements I W, Roberts F B (eds) Family health: a theoretical approach to nursing care. John Wiley, New York

Roper N, Logan W, Tierney A 2002 The elements of nursing, 4th edn. Churchill Livingstone, Edinburgh

Watson J 1999 Postmodern nursing and beyond. Churchill Livingstone, Edinburgh

4

Academic Work

❝ I haven't had to write a paper since school!'

'I had to take the Access course and although it really gave me a lot, I was still really intimidated by the kinds of assignments I had to do in the nursing course. I worked really hard on them, and did well – a lot better than I thought I would do. I've just finished my course and I'm starting my community nurse job. My advice to a new student? Don't put things off, and get support from your tutors. You'll do just fine. ❞

Jane (who was 34 when she started her nursing course)

This will be a dull, boring chapter. It is filled with little details that, although useful, are not very inspiring. But I can promise you that they will help you get better grades. Trust me.

REFERENCING

❝ An excellent paper, which would have been worthy of an A if not so poorly referenced. ❞

Feedback on a paper graded 'C'

Referencing properly does a number of things for your work. It shows:

- how widely you have read
- how critically you have looked at ideas and concepts
- that you can follow directions
- that you give credit properly to others for their ideas and work.

Students often find that poor referencing is an easy way to lose grades. You will work really hard, finding sources, making them work together ... then lose a mark because references weren't written out just the way the university wants them! Some hints:

- You will find yourself using the same sources over and over in many different modules, so keep your reference lists from all your assignments. Make sure your references are accurate and complete.
- Get, and keep, a copy of your university's referencing guidelines.
- Whenever possible, use references your instructor refers to in lectures and gives you in handouts. When they use them in their lectures, they are telling you that they value them and the information in them. How much more of a hint could that be? One thing though – they probably know those references inside out.

What doesn't need to be referenced?

There are some things that don't need to be referenced:

- common knowledge, e.g. grass is green
- undisputed facts, e.g. David Beckham was captain of the England team that played in the 2002 world cup, or Frank Skinner is a Baggies fan.

What does need to be referenced?

Things that *do* need to be referenced are:

- A quote or ideas summarized or paraphrased and taken from another text or source such as an internet page.

- Statistics, figures, diagrams or other visuals taken from any other work. Those generated as a result of the work you have done yourself in your paper don't need to be referenced.
- Things that could be challenged, e.g. 'inflation decreased last year'. A reference gives proof that your information is accurately reported (Don't take it for granted that just because it was published it is correct. A reference tells the reader you are being accurate: your arguments in the paper tell them you are right!).

Your university or nursing programme will tell you about the type of referencing it expects you to use. If you need more information, you can check on the internet by searching for 'how to reference' or for the specific reference style, e.g. 'Harvard referencing' on a search engine (www.yahoo.com is an easy one). You can also get a study guide. There is a list of suggested sources in the Useful Books, Journals and Other Resources chapter at the end of this book.

PLAGIARISM

> ⟨ Due to cheating by plagiarism, the university has no choice but to exclude you from your course. This action will be reported to the Student Grants Unit and to the English National Board... ⟩
>
> *From a letter to a student who submitted*
> *an essay purchased on the internet*

Your credibility is on the line when you write a paper. You must make sure you are being fair and honest – dishonesty can cost you, not just in grades but possibly even your place in your course and your nursing career.

The word 'plagiarism' comes from the Latin word 'plagium', which means 'kidnapper'
(Pickett et al 2000).

If I had made the above statement without a citation, you might say 'How does she know that?' You would have a right to ask!

Finding out I don't speak Latin, you would wonder:

- Is that the truth or did she just make it up?
- Did she look it up but isn't saying she did because she wants me to think she knows a lot?
- Was she was too lazy to write down where it came from?

Is that how you want your markers to be looking at your work and exams? I expect you would rather let them know that you are intelligent *and* that you are fair and honest. And plagiarism is *theft*. In most universities, plagiarism will get you thrown off the course on the first occurrence; it is an extremely serious academic offence. No matter how stressed you are, no matter how appealing 'www.buy-your-assignment-here.com' looks, it is not worth the risk.

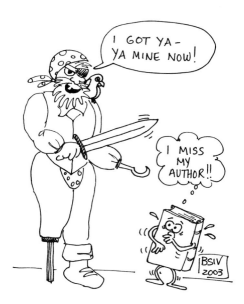

Many people who plagiarize do it unintentionally:

- They might think that they only need to cite something if they quote it directly.
- They might lose information about a source and include the information anyway (but is that titbit of information worth failing your entire assignment or exam?).

● They might have worked closely with another student and shared information and ideas (you must show that you did your work independently!).

In any case, there will be no excuse if you are found to have plagiarized something. I represented a student recently at a disciplinary hearing. She had worked with her university roommate on a particularly difficult paper. Only her roommate had gone for a tutorial and had shared her notes with her friend who had missed the class. The tutor who read both papers noticed right away that they were similar: the same references, the same concepts and the same topic. Although the students openly admitted they had worked together, each claimed that she had written her own paper. The university disagreed, and both students failed the module. They were given written warnings and had to repeat the assessment. What seemed like a good work-saver cost them the chance for a first class honours degree; it could have cost them their careers in nursing.

If you are unsure of what needs to be cited and what doesn't, ask your tutor or someone in your university's academic resource centre or library. Personally, I have cited things that I didn't really need to just to give extra weight to my argument and to be certain that there was no chance I could be accused of cheating.

WRITING AN ASSIGNMENT

❛ I keep telling myself, get it done, get it done – but I always find myself in a panic the weekend before it is due trying to write a huge assignment. This is hell! Why do I keep doing this to myself? ❜

Excerpt from a student nurse's reflective diary

In my experience, most students fail assignments because of one of three things:

● They submit a beautifully written, well thought out essay that unfortunately doesn't answer the question the assignment brief asked!

- They have rushed to do the assignment at the last minute and haven't had time to proofread it and polish it up.
- They don't know how to structure an assignment.

Answering the question

The only way to make sure you are answering the right question is to ask for a tutorial. It won't do you any good to have a tutorial before you have an idea of what you will be writing about. Try to bring a basic outline with you and always write down ideas. As soon as you walk out of the office you will forget most of what was said – write it down! An assignment brief should include:

- the title of the assignment
- a list of suggested topics (usually)
- a description of the purpose of the paper
- the word limit
- the deadline and submission information
- learning outcomes
- a marking matrix (sometimes but not always).

Sometimes, there is a topic you are really interested in that isn't one of the suggested topics. You may want to ask your marker if you can do this topic instead of one of those listed. There are pros and cons for doing this:

Pros:

- doing a unique topic can sometimes show you are innovative and creative
- a marker who has just read 60 essays on one topic might be relieved to find that essay 61 is unique
- it's always more fun to do something that you are interested in.

Cons:

- the marker may be looking for proof that you have achieved certain outcomes and your topic might not show the right kind of proof

- the marker may have a bias towards a particular perspective or approach to topics
- the marker may feel that you haven't followed the assignment brief
- something that was interesting might fade a bit after writing a comprehensive assignment about it.

How do you get around the cons? First, always discuss the choice of topics with the tutor. If you negotiate for an original topic, get it in writing!

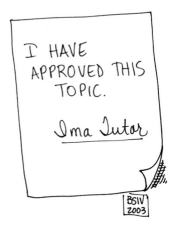

The information you are given in class will also guide you to what is expected from the assignment. If you are being given information about certain models, theories or concepts, the marker will probably expect to see them in your assignment.

Make sure you understand the question. I know a nursing student who wrote an assignment on incontinence for a module called 'Care of the chronically ill'. She had beautiful graphs and charts, discussed different care products, discussed an incontinence assessment, outlined the complications of incontinence, the causes of incontinence, looked at the patient holistically, had good references and presented the assignment flawlessly. She failed. The problem? The assignment brief listed 'will discuss the nursing management of a group of patients with this need' and 'will reflect upon the work of the nursing team in improving patient outcomes'. Her paper talked a lot about the problem but didn't touch on those learning outcomes. When you finish your paper, read it through and check off elements that meet the learning outcomes. Make sure you have them all covered.

Some modules may give you a marking matrix. This should tell you all the elements expected in the assignment and how heavily they will be weighted.

You should also consider the level at which you are doing the assignment. Common foundation work is usually assessed at a lower standard than Branch, and work at bachelor's degree is higher than work at diploma. The higher the academic level, the more you will be expected to challenge and be critical (questioning) about what you see and learn (see the academic levels table in the appendix at the end of the chapter).

Timing it right

You need to plan a time frame for your paper. Use your diary or a calendar to plan out deadlines for the different stages of your assignment. My suggestion is that you:

- Write in your diary the date the paper is due. Then, back-track a week and write it in again as due. Try to get it done by the earlier date.
- Make deadlines for yourself: when the first draft will be done, when your tutorial will be, etc. Stick to them.
- Save all your work on *two* disks as well as on your computer. Floppy disks can fail. Don't save anything on a university or shared computer. One way to back-up is to e-mail yourself your assignment!

Structuring your assignment

Every assignment you write should have four main parts:

1. **The introduction:** you use this section to tell the reader what is coming. Using your module guide, assignment guide and marking matrix, map out what you are going to talk about. Try to have a logical flow from one area of discussion to another.
2. **The body:** in this part, you follow the pattern set in the introduction. Link paragraphs logically, and watch your continuity.
3. **The conclusion:** this is where you summarize everything else, and reaffirm that you have covered what you promised to cover.
4. **The reference list:** the sources you cited in the paper.

A mistake many students make is not organizing their information properly. This book is too small for me to explain in detail, but try to follow a map when you are writing your papers – don't jump around but have information follow logically. Don't worry if you aren't a great writer – having good flow and good writing styles will get you good grades but you don't need to be Charlotte Brontë to pass.

Another mistake many students make is writing in the wrong 'voice'. Some of the reference papers you read as background will be in an academic style, which means that instead of saying (for example) 'I agree …', the author must say 'this student agrees …' or 'the author agrees …'. Informal writing, or narrative writing allows the author to 'speak' in first tense. This book is written in narrative style – as though I am talking to you. Make sure you know what 'voice' your tutor wants for the paper. Usually, reflections can be done in a narrative voice but everything else needs to be in academic voice.

Preparing for your assignment

There is a lot you must do to prepare for your academic assignment:

- **Know what is expected of you:** what the question is that the assignment is answering and the format expected of the completed work.

- **Research your sources.**
- Have a referencing guide to make sure your references are done properly.
- Have a study guide book to help you map out, plan and complete your assignments.
- **Leave enough time to do your work.** Although assignments done at the last minute can be successful, they are hell on your spirit, your sense of humour and the bags under your eyes. Get it done sooner and be lounging about with a pint in the student union bar while your friends are panicking.

If you leave it until the night before to type up your assignment, I can guarantee that some of the following will happen:

- Your computer will crash, eating all but eight words of your 3000-word assignment on wound care, just as a burglar breaks into your house and steals your only back-up copy.
- You will run out of paper, ink, electricity and/or brain cells.
- You will oversleep and pass the assignment in 4 minutes after the deadline.
- Your sister will break up with her fiancée and spend all evening sitting in your room, eating chocolate chunk ice cream and crying all over you.
- You will meet the perfect partner and have to choose between writing about the joys of leg ulcer care or jetting off to a holiday in Crete.
- Your two best friends from the course will have done the same thing and be on the phone to you in a panic begging to work together.
- Your friend who did her work early will be gloating at you from her seat in the student union bar ...

When you get your assignment back ...

- Look at the feedback and look through the paper for any notes or comments. Use the feedback to guide the way you write other papers. If you disagree strongly with any of the comments, bring them to the marker's attention.

- Keep the assignment. It has information in it that has already been critiqued. It could be useful for other work!

If you do particularly poorly on an assignment, make an appointment to speak to the tutor. Ask to review the marked copy of the paper. Make a note of the points raised so you can do better next time.

Always book an appointment for tutorial help. Dropping in might look easier but neither you nor the tutor is really ready and it won't be the best use of anyone's time. Don't wait – book your tutorial early to make sure you get one. If you struggle to write assignments, get a tutorial from your university's student support services, ask the student union if they have workshops on assignment writing, ask another student for help, approach a tutor and ask for help, or look at one of the books listed in the Useful Books, Journals and Other Resources chapter at the end of this book.

Some final points: don't leave your assignments lying around; don't leave them on the 'desktop' of uni computers; don't give them to other people (who may copy them). You are working really hard; don't let someone steal your hard work. If two people hand in similar assignments, it will be noticed and both parties could be called before a Cheating Board. Make your life simple: keep your assignments to yourself.

CONFIDENTIALITY AND PRIVACY

❛ I was in the lift talking about my patient to my friend on the course. I didn't say his name or anything, so I thought it was OK. Later, a lady who had been in the lift with us came to visit my patient. The look on the visitor's face said it all when she saw me. I felt dreadful. ❜

First year nursing student

As a student nurse, and continuing as a nurse, you will have access to sensitive and personal information about patients and their families. They may be your friends, your neighbours, well known people or people who are in particularly delicate circumstances. You have an obligation to keep that information private. If you fail to maintain confidentiality, your patients could suffer and so will your grades. You could even find yourself excluded from the course.

Always blank-out the name of hospitals and wards on documents you put into any written assignment – you should never refer to any trust or facility by name. Instead of 'Clipper 1, the Gynaecology Ward at Smythfields NHS Trust' you should put 'On a gynaecology ward of a local trust'. Community hospitals serve people who live and work locally. It wouldn't be hard to for someone to (correctly or incorrectly) work out that their 42-year-old neighbour who was recently in the hospital could be the 42-year-old man suffering from alcohol withdrawal who was discussed in your paper, especially if he lives in the same area as the hospital you mentioned. Again, it's not just ethics at risk here, it's your grades. You will lose marks if you don't handle information sensitively and professionally.

You also have to be careful about the manner in which you refer to patients. Being judgemental makes you look unprofessional. How would you feel about each of the following statements?

> 'The patient was abusive and rude, and staff had to force him to wash. His smell offended other patients, probably because he slept rough. He was a filthy mess but his skin was OK.'
>
> or
>
> 'The patient had a long history of alcoholism and had been homeless for some time. He appeared distressed and upset. His hygiene was poor, so staff assisted him in bathing. Skin and nutritional assessments were done.'

Those two paragraphs say the same thing about the patient – but different things about the nurses who wrote them. Being unprofessional will cost you marks. It also shows your lack of fitness to be a nurse.

The NMC *Guidelines for Records and Record Keeping* are repro-duced in Chapter 11 (see p. 192) – get to know them and follow them. Although they don't specifically mention confidentiality in written academic assignments, they do discuss being judgemental.

There are some important points that you must remember about patient privacy and written assignments:

- You must ask permission from patients if you are using them as a case study or will be referring to them in your paper or documentation for your university.
- You must change identifying information about them so no one can tell who they are by your description.
- Note in your paper that you are using a pseudonym (cite it – show you know the rules!).
- Never identify the ward, trust or area in which you cared for the patient except in general terms.
- You must be professional in your descriptions and observa-tions, never judgemental or biased.

Also, never refer to classmates or work colleagues by name in your papers. It is an issue of privacy for them, too. How would you feel if one of your classmates referred to you by name? Always keep details of everyone – the trust, the staff, the patients – confidential.

BASIC IT SKILLS

Which are you?

A I remember when calculators first came out. They were big, bulky and expensive. I still use a slide rule. I hated technology then and I hate it now. I write my assignments in pencil.

B I have a computer. I don't know what kind, but it has Office on it.

C My computer is a Pentium 26z with 4096 gig of RAM, a CD-RW, a DVD player, surround-sound speakers, a built-in microwave, seating for ten and a panoramic webview of the Edgbaston cricket ground.

Whichever you are, you will probably need to use a computer during your nurse education:

- to write assignments
- to research information on the internet and in the library
- to use study materials found on CD
- to play games when you are so stressed you want to run away from home
- to e-mail family and friends who are not on your course to tell them that although they haven't seen or heard from you in weeks, you are still alive, just working on an assignment
- on placements for patient details and records.

Most universities have tutorials on computer usage. If you are:

- Person A: go; don't be afraid. Computers are (usually) pretty easy to use and, with the right support, you will be able to build skills and confidence.
- Person B: go; you will build confidence and learn easier ways to do things you already know how to do.
- Person C: go; you will be a support to your friends and classmates. Don't be tempted to do all their work online for them – you won't have time to get your own done if your friends all look to you as the resident net guru.

If your university or nursing programme does *not* have IT tutorials, find out why! It should be preparing you to use computers as part of your eventual work as a nurse.

If you don't have a computer or internet access, your university should have a computer room with access. Remember to take your own floppy disks to save information on and don't forget that in peak times (when assignments are due) it could be very difficult to access a computer. Plan ahead.

There are some great books that can help you with using different computer programs – I love the … *For Dummies* books. Even as an experienced computer user (Yes, sadly I am person 'C'), I find them useful.

Other resources can be found in your library. Useful search engines, such as Ovid and the British Nursing Index (BNI), catalogue periodicals. Some online resources and databases that you can access from home or university require you to have an 'Athens' password. They are free to students who have registered through their university. Speak to the librarian or IT helpdesk to find out how to get access to Ovid, the BNI, CINAHL, and how to get an Athens password.

See if there is information on 'how to search'. It may sound simple but knowing how to search properly is a very valuable skill. Some learning resource centres run short courses to help you gain confidence in searching. It's a good investment. Although there is a little about literature searches in Chapter 9, it is too vast a skill for me to teach you here. Your learning resource centre/university library is the best place to start if you need to learn to search for sources and information. A short list of resource books appears in the Useful Books, Journals and Other Resources chapter at the end of this book.

REFERENCES

Pickett J et al (eds) 2000 The American heritage dictionary of the English language, 4th edn. Houghton Mifflin, Boston

APPENDIX 4.1: ACADEMIC LEVELS

Level	Who is at this level?	What is expected of them?
1	Most CFP students, most 1st- and some 2nd-year students in degree or diploma courses	Starting to develop skills, explores different ideas and concepts; shows awareness of different ideas; basic skills in presenting and preparing academic work
2	2nd-year degree students, 3rd-year diploma students, some post-registration courses	Building on level 1. Able to show further development of skills; shows a greater understanding of issues and topics; observes and reflects on

(continued)

Level	Who is at this level?	What is expected of them?
		events; demonstrates the ability to analyse information; shows greater exploration and recognition of issues, topics and ideas
3	3rd-/4th-year degree, some 3rd-year diploma, some post-registration courses	Shows synthesis of knowledge and skills. Able to use analysis and critical evaluation; investigates and evaluates theories, ideas and information; uses reflection to improve practice and to build awareness; able to understand theoretical–practical links and relevance
4	Master's level	As other levels but with greater depth and with original thought and understanding. Study at this level requires personal motivation, being able to look at past works and generate original concepts and ideas. At this level, nurses are expected to be making themselves available to others as expert practitioners
	Doctorate level	As other levels, but with specific expertise in specialty area

Clinical Placements

5

❝ On my first placement, I was walking through the ward and I heard a patient cry out "Nurse! Nurse!" Suddenly, I realized she meant ME! – I was the nurse! ❞
Student nurse reflective diary

❝ I'd been a health care assistant before, so I knew how to get people washed and dressed, but it took me a while to start thinking differently. I had to stop thinking like an HCA so I could become a nurse. ❞
Third year student nurse

In this chapter

There have been enormous changes in the NHS over the last 20 years. This chapter concentrates on those that affect nurse education and Appendix 6 outlines Agenda for Change – the most recent changes to the grading, promotion and payment of nurses.

PROJECT 2000

Nurse education has changed dramatically since the 1980s. Once, nursing students were employed by hospitals as apprentices.

They were educated in the hospital; they worked on and staffed the wards. They learned everything through experience. These students often had the same responsibilities and demands placed on them as the staff nurses. It would not have been uncommon to go onto a ward and find a senior student supervising junior students, with no sign of a staff nurse anywhere.

However, it was decided that nurse education had to become more academically based. Nurses had good skills but not enough theory or evidence to help them progress as things changed. In 1989/1990, Project 2000 was introduced. This took what had formerly been called 'pupil' or 'apprentice' nurses and made them into students, and not just in name – it took the base for training nurses out of the clinical areas and moved to it to universities.

There were some radical changes: nursing students would now be supernumary, where previously they were used to help staff clinical areas. They would receive an education to prepare them both academically and clinically. They would have the benefits and support that come with being a full-time student.

Although this change was heralded by many as the most significant ever to have occurred in nurse education, some people were really very worried that it was the death knell for competent clinical practice. In 1999, the Department of Health (DoH) admitted that, in many ways, Project 2000 was not meeting the needs of the modern NHS. In part, this finding was based on the Peach report.

THE PEACH REPORT

The Peach report – also called *Fitness for Practice* (UKCC 1999) – looked at the nature of nurse education and made recommendations to 'prepare a way forward for pre-registration nursing and midwifery education that enable fitness for practice based on health care need' (UKCC 1999 p. 2). The recommendations provided guidance for making nursing students into nurses who were fit for practice and fit for purpose.

Recommendation 10 in the Peach report states that 'consistent clinical supervision in a supportive learning environment during all practice placements is necessary' (p. 37) and a number of recommendations suggest that higher education institutes and service providers (trusts, placement areas, etc.) should work together to provide the best education for students (UKCC 1999).

MAKING A DIFFERENCE

Following the Peach report, the DoH published *Making a Difference* (DoH 1999). This set out a number of priorities for nurse education:

- There needed to be flexible career pathways into and through nurse and midwifery education.
- There needed to be an increased emphasis on practice within the educational programme.
- The educational programme needed to be more responsive to the needs of the modern NHS.

Making a Difference was published in 1999, and further consultations with the UKCC (the forerunner of the NMC) set out the changes that would be made to pre-registration nurse education. These changes included:

- step-on/step-off points
- part-time and more flexible programmes
- cadet schemes
- better links between vocational training and nurse education to help people make their way into nurse education in later life
- better, longer clinical placements
- a stronger role for the NHS in choosing students.

Despite these changes, one thing that did not change was the Branch structure.

THE BRANCHES OF NURSING

The Peach report (UKCC 1999) also recommended a review of the current Branch structure of nurse education. As discussed in Chapter 1, there are currently four branches in pre-registration nurse education – adult nurse, children's nurse, mental health nurse and learning disability nurse. Whereas Peach (UKCC 1999) suggested that the Branches needed to be reviewed, many other people have suggested that a return to 'generalist' education is needed. The UK is the only country in the world to separate nurse education into these four Branches, and this makes it difficult for nurses qualified in a Branch other than adult nursing to register and work in other countries. However, nurses in the Branches other than adult nursing feel that they have been specially prepared to care for vulnerable specialized patients. This will be an ongoing issue.

You will have placements in your own area of nursing. In addition, you will probably have a placement in three of the following areas (not including your own Branch) to familiarize you with the different Branches:

- child health
- learning disability
- mental health nursing
- maternal health
- adult nursing.

Placements can be in a number of different areas and formats:

- public-sector hospital, care home, GP practice, or other facility
- private-sector hospital, care home, or other facility
- in a school, nursery or with school nurse
- in the community with health visitors or district nurses
- independently arranged (electives) in which students find the area in which they wish to take a placement
- private study (usually done with a workbook or to produce a piece of academic work that reviews a clinical area)

- overseas placements and electives – these can be very complicated to arrange, as well as expensive, so if you are interested in going to another country for a placement, speak to your personal tutor and the allocations department, and look for funding as soon as you can; if you wait, the placement might not be possible. The Royal College of Nursing has written some helpful guidance on overseas placements for nursing students.

Because of the increasing number of nursing students it can be very difficult for the university to place all the students within a certain geographical area. This means that more and more nursing students are finding that they need to travel quite long distances to their placements, or that they are being given an alternative placement such as private study. It also means that mentors and staff nurses in clinical areas are often stretched to provide the supervision and support that student nurses need.

So, what does this mean to you on placement?

CLINICAL PLACEMENTS

Your placements will take place in different areas and usually in different trusts. You will be relying on staff nurses and other staff members (such as physiotherapists, doctors) to help meet your learning outcomes and gain the experience you need to become a qualified nurse.

A few things to remember:

- **Patients have the right to say no to having a student care for them:** when you introduce yourself, tell the patient you are a student and make sure you have their permission. Don't assume.
- **You have more to prove than any other member of staff:** dress and look the part of an eager and well-prepared student. Clean, appropriate uniform and appearance will score you immeasurable points with staff and patients alike. Staff will

be looking at you critically – don't give them any cause to doubt you.

- **Nail varnish and make-up:** can be vectors for infection (i.e. carry infective material that can get into a patient's wounds) and **cologne, perfume and make-up** can all be allergens. People with allergies and breathing difficulties can be made very ill by exposure to some make-up and cologne. Don't use them on placements.
- **Rings, bracelets and long fingernails:** these can scratch patients and can be vectors for infection. Don't wear them. You might lose them or ruin them anyway.
- **If your hair is long, tie it back:** this is as much for your safety as it is for cleanliness.
- **Necklaces and chains around the neck, and earrings, facial studs, etc.:** these can be dangerous – confused or aggressive patients could grab and pull them.

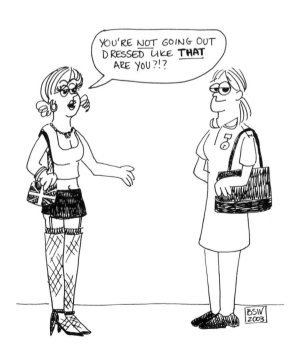

- **Uniforms:** if the uni says wear grey trousers, wear grey trousers. Wear your uniform according to the university policy. If you wear mufti (street clothes) make sure you are dressed appropriately. Football strips, tee-shirts with slogans, and stained or torn clothing all say 'I'm not very professional' and could upset vulnerable patients.
- **BE ON TIME.**
- **Visit the placement in advance:** when you find out the time and location of your placement, call and make an appointment to visit. Try to meet your mentor and/or some of the ward staff. Ask about shifts, parking, where to put your coat, if you need to bring your own cup/teabags, etc. Find out about the off duty (when you are working).
- **Know what happens in the placement area:** when you are scheduled for a particular placement area, prepare yourself. Don't be like a Miss America student who, when asked what she would like, said 'A general overview. And world peace'. Be specific. Think about the kinds of specialties and patients the ward will have, think about what interests you in the specialty and ask about it. Try to prepare for special terms! For example, if it's an ear nose and throat (ENT) ward, get an ENT textbook out of the library, brush up on the anatomy and physiology of the ear, nose and throat, and try to learn some of the terms you will encounter. The nurses and staff there will have invested a lot in their specialty and seeing a student motivated to learn about their kind of nursing will inspire them. That means a better placement for you.
- **Develop student 'antennae':** try to work out the best – and worst – times to approach your mentor or other staff nurses. It makes life easier for everyone – especially you. Just imagine … you are driving to work in the lovely brand new car you and your partner have saved so hard to buy. As the result of some rather unfortunate experiences, by the time you get home the car looks more like a piece of modern art than the beautiful new car you set off in this morning: it's a write-off. Your partner comes home, an hour late, looking rather flustered and

upset – bad day at the office. Now you have a grouchy, frustrated partner who is on and off the phone trying to solve a complicated problem. Is this the best moment to say 'Darling, I crashed the car?' No, it's the best time to help your partner get through the crisis and then, when it's over, you can explain how you have a submission for the Turner Prize called 'Was once a car …' and how your partner now has a perfect opportunity to buy that other model he or she wanted. It's the same with your mentor.

- **Be sensitive to patient perspectives:** patients will sometimes do or say things that really aren't acceptable in our culture. Ridiculously biased things like 'I don't want a black nurse', 'You're too fat to be my nurse' or 'I don't want a male nurse, they're all gay'. Please, don't allow yourself to be abused but try to remember that when people are ill they aren't themselves. Some patients will have wandering hands. Try not to over-react or be afraid. Be firm but caring. Remember that your appearance can sometimes seem threatening to some patients. If you have brightly dyed hair, a lot of facial piercings, and/or visible tattoos, there is a chance that some patients could react. I have even had people react to my American accent! They said things that were hurtful, although they didn't intend them to be that way. People who are ill are afraid, and people who are afraid often cope in very strange ways. If someone slips up and says something unkind or judgemental, they are not reacting to you as a person: it's up to you to try to be therapeutic anyway. If someone abuses you, get support from your mentor and other nurses.

- **Be sensitive to staff too:** be aware of and respect policies, procedures and chain of command in the area in which you are working. Try to think of yourself as an ambassador – your behaviour and attitude will affect the way future nursing students are treated. One student can ruin it for all the other students who follow and can make things very difficult for staff. Do the best you can to respect the way staff do things.

We'll talk more about things as the chapter goes on, but if you remember nothing else, remember this:

Always be on time, neat, clean and dressed appropriately to make the best, most professional impression.

What kind of student are you?

You're probably tired of talking about nursing and placements, so let's take a minute to talk about something else…

Let's imagine that you are going on a wonderful holiday. You have been given a week-long adventure in Florida. You have been to a travel agent, who has given you a list of all the places you can visit. You have been told you will have a dedicated tour guide while you are there. You are leaving in 3 weeks. What do you do?

A   You wait for the tour guide to send you info, and aren't particularly bothered when they don't.

B   You ask friends who have been to Florida about their experiences.

C   You get brochures and maybe even a book to give you more information about the sights and ideas about what to do.

Your cases are packed and you are on your way. You get to your hotel, unpack and wait for your tour guide to show up. The office says that they are overbooked, so the tour guide is not coming today. In fact, they can't tell you when or if the tour guide is ever going to come. Do you:

A   Sit by the pool, not worrying that you only have a week and have a lot of things you would like to do.

B   Try to get something done that is on your list.

C   Call the travel agent and let them know that there is a problem.

The travel agent calls you and asks how things are going. You explain the tour guide situation and the agent tells you to go it alone today while he or she tries to do something for you. Do you:

A Do nothing but get a sunburn waiting for someone to call you back.

B Do something around the hotel – maybe EastEnders is on TV!

C Do something nearby that is on your list.

Your tour guide, as a result of a short call from your travel agency, shows up the next day. She asks you what you would like to do. Do you:

A Shrug your shoulders and say 'I dunno'.

B Say 'Whatever you want me to will be OK with me'.

C Grab your pamphlets and books and point out what interests you.

Your tour guide takes you to two places that day – one is really naff and the other is the most wonderful and amazing place you have ever seen. The next day, when you have some free time, do you …

A Complain to everyone about what kind of experience you had at the naff place.

B Talk about how great the good place was.

C Write about the good place – you want to remember all the details!

At the end of the holiday, you have had a great time. There are some people who really made a difference to you. The tour guide, once she showed up, was pretty amazing and really gave a lot extra. The clerk at the hotel was very friendly. Even the housekeeper treated you like her own child. What do you do?

A Leave a mess – after all they are paid to clean up after you, and mumble something that sounds like 'Thanks' as the taxi comes to take you to the airport.

B   Think about how great everyone has been.

C   Thank each person, and send a card to the hotel manager and tour guide agency telling them how good the experience was.

Your plane lands and you are walking through the airport. Everyone seems to be looking at you and there are television cameras; people are taking your picture. It seems your trip was part of a new reality television show ...

Looking back, were you the 'A' tourist – the one who waited for every experience to be inflicted on them, who complained, and who had no initiative? Or were you the 'B' tourist – the one who made some effort but didn't do much work? Or were you the 'C' tourist – the one who planned ahead, had initiative, showed real gratitude and who took control of the holiday? The prize for the best contestant was a passing grade ... which of the three tourists do you think would win that coveted pass?

OK, a bit of fun, but in reality the difference between a naff clinical placement and a good one isn't really the mentor, the placement or even the other staff. It's all in how *you*, the student, approaches what's before you. It's *your* placement.

What if things go wrong?

You have a number of options when there are problems on your placement:

- ignore them and hope they go away
- avoid them by calling in sick
- keep your head down and try just to live through it
- complain to everyone who will listen
- go to your university or the ward manager (or the clinical placement facilitator) and explain the problem, asking for help and support.

The sooner you flag a problem or ask for help, the more likely there is to be a good outcome for you. If you wait until you get your final assessment to complain about your mentor, it will look like you are trying to get out of a bad review and it's unlikely you will be taken seriously.

In the unlikely event that things start to go wrong, you need to do a few things:

- **Document!** Write down when things are said or done that aren't right. Keep a time line – when things happened, who did them, etc. Don't be in the situation where you have to say 'I don't know who told me, but …'
- **Reflect: what is really going wrong?** Is any of it your fault? Did you make things worse? What do you need to do differently? What do you need to go forward?
- **Make sure of the rules.** Check policies and university guidelines. Is it your perspective that is wrong or is something being done improperly?

If you do need to complain, you have to know how:

- **Take an advocate:** your union, student union or university rep should be with you. Talk to him or her – they are used to complaining and sorting things out.
- Use your time line to show a clear history of the problem.
- **Be objective:** don't get personal. 'She hates me' is not a good place to start a complaint. Relate specific examples openly and honestly.
- **Be willing to work things out:** don't get stubborn or difficult. Express what is wrong, what you need, and try to be flexible.
- **Let go of the past:** if things are discussed and everyone makes plans to move forward, don't hold a grudge. Be a professional and be willing to give others a chance.

To summarize all this, remember: this is *your* placement. Your mentor, the ward manager and the other staff nurses already passed their course. It's not up to you to worry about them, it's up to you to worry about you. If they don't do things the right way then learn from their example anyway. You can learn from bad practice just as you can learn from good practice.

You may find yourself in a situation where you witness something you cannot ignore: a medication error, harm to a patient, theft, abuse. If that is the case, seek support from someone before bringing it forward. As a student, you are vulnerable and you must accept that there are times when you need support. Whistle blowing is a serious issue and can be very stressful. You are obliged to blow the whistle if you witness something serious, and there are people at your university and in your union who are obliged to help you. Don't feel you have to go it alone. I can't really prepare you here for the stress and anxiety that whistle-blowing could potentially bring – if you know that something must be brought out into the open, get support through your uni, union or student union.

SUPERNUMARY STATUS

❛ I know students are supposed to be supernumary, but how are they going to learn to be nurses if they sit at the desk reading a magazine? ❜

Mentor

Supernumary status is one of those things that has no real definition. What it means in theory is that you are not staff on the ward so you do not have the same responsibilities and obligations. Whereas other staff are there to take care of patients and meet the needs of the ward, you are there to meet your learning needs and objectives. This can conflict with the nature of clinical placements. On placement, you learn by 'being a nurse', by giving hands-on care and by pitching in as part of the team. There is a subtle but important difference – you:

- are there to learn
- must be supervised
- are there to help out as a team member to learn about the team and how it works

- must meet your learning outcomes
- must stay within the scope of your knowledge and skills as a student nurse.

You are not:

- there to staff the ward
- there to fulfil the role of any other nurse or nursing assistant in their absence
- there to supervise any patient in a one-to-one capacity (because you yourself need supervision)
- to put 'getting the work done' before your learning
- ever to step beyond the limitations of your role, no matter what you know from your past career and education
- to 'cover' the placement area without a nurse present.

It is difficult – the ward is down a nurse and a healthcare assistant and the patients are still in bed at 10.00 a.m. You want to go to see a diagnostic test being done on a patient you have been following all week. The sister tells you that you are needed to bathe patients and so you can't go. What do you do? There is no easy answer.

An isolated episode like this doesn't mean your supernumary status has been compromised. I hope you never stand on a ward with your hands on your hips while patients are in need and say, 'I'm a student and I am not going to help'. You have to use your judgement. If it is happening all the time or you hear 'We don't need a health-care assistant, we have a student …' then do something about it:

- document what is happening
- talk to the ward manager, your mentor, the university and your union as soon as you are aware of the problem
- don't just ignore it – other students, and most important, patients – are affected.

So, points to remember about being supernumary … Being super-numary means:

- you are not there to replace, or to fill in for, a member of staff at any level

- you need to put your learning outcomes before the staffing needs of the placement area
- you do have a role as a member of the team on the placement area
- you have a responsibility to patients and families
- you must never act outside the scope of your education and student role
- you have the right to mentorship and support in meeting your learning outcomes
- you are *not* a nurse and you are *not* a healthcare assistant – you are a student who is there to learn while doing and to practice essential skills to gain competency.

Ask yourself: Is this helping me become a good, competent nurse? Am I learning new skills and building on established ones? Am I getting chances to have new experiences and to grow as a nurse? If the answer is 'Yes' then you are probably OK.

MENTORSHIP

When you start a placement, you will be assigned a mentor. This person assesses you and will sign-off your competencies. They will usually have undertaken a mentorship and assessors course.

If you plan a pre-placement visit to the placement area, you really should try to meet your mentor. You will probably follow a similar off duty (work schedule) as your mentor to make sure you have ample time to work together. You should work with your mentor at least two shifts a week. Busy placement areas will often assign you one mentor and a 'back-up' mentor, so that you have the best support, and to take the pressure off staff. Your mentor is there to:

- make sure you meet the required competencies to pass the placement
- be your teacher and supervisor

- make certain you comply with policies like manual handling
- fulfil the requirement that someone qualified to be a mentor is present in placement areas where there are students.

Your mentor is also there to do a number of other things:

- staff the ward
- do paperwork
- take care of patients
- take care of families
- resolve complaints and staff issues
- do the off duty
- answer the phone
- pass medications
- do treatments and dressings
- monitor patients
- respond to consultants' and doctors' requests and orders
- do care planning …

… I'm sure you get the hint – your mentor is a busy nurse. Often, your mentor will be a ward sister (or charge nurse), the busiest of all the ward nurses on any given shift. How can you and this nurse make the best of this important relationship?

- **Have a clue:** go into your placement knowing what you need to accomplish and have some idea of how you plan to accomplish your goals and outcomes. Read about the placement area before you go in. What kind of nursing is it? What kinds of patients will there be?
- **Be a good team member:** respect the fact that sister (or the charge nurse) may have pressing things to accomplish. Don't wait for her to approve your every move – the rest of the team from domestic to HCA to staff nurse all have knowledge you can make use of. Build a good network for yourself.
- **Know the deadlines:** be assertive about getting your paperwork done. 'Sister, I need my assessment done by Friday. Can we

schedule some time please? I've already done my part ...'
Don't wait for her or him to psychically determine that you
are ready for your assessment. It's *your* assessment, *you* need
to make sure it gets done. Don't wait until the end of your
placement – make sure your assessments are done when they
are due.

- **Communicate:** tell your mentor or other staff nurse when you
are having problems. Ask for help when you need it. Let someone know if something is going wrong as soon as possible. You
have a lot of resources – union reps, student union, placement
facilitators, uni staff, personal tutors, ward managers: if something is going wrong and you don't tell anyone, it is no one's
fault but yours when your mentor fails you.

- **Get along:** not everyone is compatible with everyone else.
You will have mentors who don't like you and you will have
mentors you don't like. You might not agree with them, you
might just be so different as individuals that you can't see
eye to eye. Be professional and do the best you can to get
along. This doesn't mean you should allow yourself to be
bullied or mistreated, it just means that you shouldn't expect
every mentor to be your best friend. Learning to get along
with different kinds of people is essential to nursing: it's
yet another lesson you can learn from your student–mentor
relationship.

- **Be professional:** don't *ever* do things you are not qualified to
do. Don't cover up mistakes. Ask for help when you need it.
Be cheerful and pleasant, and don't gossip.

- Use 'student antennae'.

Your mentor should make sure that your placement gives you
skills and experience. Sometimes that won't work quite the way
you want it to. By working cooperatively with the placement area
staff and being responsible for yourself, you give your assessment
the best foundation it can have. Ultimately, it is up to you – your
conduct, your behaviour, your skills – to make sure you pass your
placement.

Student antennae

Summary

It all boils down to AAA:

A **Attendance:** show up on time and only pull a sickie if you truly need it because you are sick.

A **Appearance:** look the part of a professional nurse.

A **Attitude:** have a smile on your face, be positive and don't complain when things go wrong – look for solutions.

If you want to be taken seriously as a professional nurse, look like one. Be:

- neat
- clean (and without excess makeup and jewellery)
- on time.

There are different Branches in nursing and you will have placements in the different Branch areas. If you decide you want to go into a different Branch, you can negotiate to change Branches. Remember that:

- Your placements are there to develop you into a competent qualified nurse.

- You need to be an active and eager participant in your education and development.
- You may need to complain, seek help or blow the whistle: know the contact details of the people who are there to help you at your union, your student union, your university and the trust in which you are placed.
- You are supernumary but that doesn't mean that you sit around waiting to be taught something; it also means that you do not replace paid staff. Being a team member is essential to learning how to be a competent nurse. You are there to get your learning outcomes met and to become more competent.
- Your mentor will be a busy nurse with many responsibilities. Be considerate and know what you need for help and support.
- Be prepared to be assertive – but also understanding – about getting your needs met.
- It's *your* placement, *your* portfolio, *your* pass. Know your portfolio and assessment documents and take responsibility for getting things done.

The next chapter is about assertiveness and the other skills essential to surviving placements and nurse education. Not skills like taking a blood pressure or passing a nasogastric tube, but skills like how to stand up for yourself!

> ❛ I'm a mentor now and every time my student nurse frustrates me, I try to think back to when I was a student. I remember being a student nurse and thinking, 'When did my mentor develop such amnesia about being a student nurse herself?' It helps me be a little more patient and understanding about how difficult it can be to be a student nurse. I just wish the student could understand how hard it can be to be a mentor! ❜
>
> *Nurse, qualified 3 years*

REFERENCES

Department of Health 1999 Making a difference. HMSO, London
UKCC 1999 Fitness for practice (the Peach report). UKCC, London

Tools of the Trade

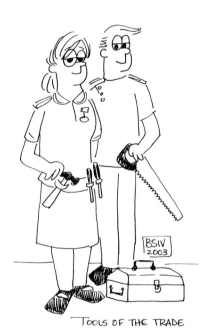

TOOLS OF THE TRADE

As a student, you will be actively developing skills from the first day you enter your course. Some of those skills will be obvious – manual handling, for example – but some of them won't be. You will be changing the way you think and act as you learn more about nursing and health care.

It is a good idea if, from the very start, you think and act with a mind towards how you want to be as a nurse. This is much easier said than done but, like any practical skill or habit, practice makes perfect.

ASSERTIVENESS

What is assertiveness?

- Respecting the rights and feelings of others while taking care of yourself.
- Standing up for yourself and your rights.
- Making clear what you want and need in a respectful way.
- Being honest with yourself and others about what you need, what you can do, and how you are feeling.
- Expressing your needs in a way that focuses on solutions.

Being assertive isn't the same as being a bully – when you behave in an assertive way, you shouldn't be hurting people's feelings or making people upset. Assertiveness doesn't include any of the following:

- blaming, shaming, name calling
- unreasonable demands
- being manipulative
- anger, shouting, violence
- gossiping, backstabbing, prejudice.

Are you assertive?

I think most people would say they struggle to be assertive, but it's really an essential skill for a good nurse. It requires practice and reflection to develop assertiveness skills.

Some common feelings can get in the way when people try to be assertive. Remember that other people feel the same as you do when they try to be assertive – even people who seem really confident and self-assured. I'm a very assertive person but sometimes I have to take a deep breath and overcome some very big butterflies in my guts when asserting myself! At some time or another, everyone feels:

- afraid that others will reject them
- afraid that they will do something stupid
- afraid of being embarrassed
- afraid of losing friends or being gossiped about.

It's not just you who feels this way! But it can be very scary to assert yourself, especially when the person you are confronting is more powerful, more knowledgeable or is aggressive. This is why you should be assertive even when it is scary:

- If you don't, you will feel upset that you didn't stand up for yourself.
- If you let people take advantage of you, they will continue until you stand up to them or they grind you down.
- If you can't take care of yourself, you can't hope to take care of anyone else (like patients!).
- Feeling used, disrespected, taken advantage of and powerless to speak up leads to stress and unhappiness.
- By asserting yourself, you could change things for the better for everyone. Chances are, you are not the only person feeling the way you do!

Of course, there are some times when you can't assert yourself. 'Excuse me, I understand that you have had a lot to drink, but would you mind putting that machete down? It's making me very nervous.' If being assertive isn't going to get you anywhere, don't do it!

How do you frame an assertive confrontation?

1. **State the problem** (remember, stick to objective explanations, no feelings, no blame, no shame).

2. State what you need and expect.
3. Show the shared value in getting a good resolution.
4. **Know your limits,** and think about what you will do if the person you are asserting yourself to won't work with you.

For example: You get the off duty and you find that you are scheduled to work the weekend. Again. This is the third weekend in a row. You go to see the person who does the off duty.

What you need to do	For example ...
State the problem	'I have seen the off duty, and I am scheduled to work this weekend. I have worked the past two weekends in a row.'
State what you need and expect	'I should have this weekend off. I believe I have done my share.'
Show the shared value	'I don't mind doing my share when I see the shifts are covered fairly.'
Know your limits	Have a plan for what to do if they don't see that having you work all the weekends is a problem: see the ward manager, talk to the union steward, etc.

The person you are confronting could respond in a number of different ways:

The response	Your reaction
'I'm sorry, I made a mistake, I'll fix it.'	'I thought it was something like that, thanks for taking care of it.' (Smile!)
'I'm sorry, I made a mistake, but it's too late to schedule someone else.	Is it worth arguing here? Either stick to your guns ('I am not working') or offer a reasonable alternative ('I'll work, but I'd like the next four weekends in a row off to make up for the weekends I have worked.')

(continued)

The response	Your reaction
'I'm the one who does the off duty, if you don't like it, tough!'	'Thank you for explaining this to me. I will need to discuss this with the ward manager.' Then, *go* to the ward manager
'No one else can work weekends, so I have to schedule you.'	'I am not able to work every weekend; I feel that it's something we all should share.' Then, go to see the ward manager and ask for help.

It's easier to handle the response you might get if you think about it in advance. In this case, you would need to know in advance what kinds of alternatives you were willing to accept. Planning for a 'win–win' scenario (where each side gets some benefit) is important in making a good assertive confrontation. Think: what are the end results that you would be willing to accept?

A few points:

- **Be positive:** smile, be calm and don't overreact.
- **Always act as if a problem is the result of a misunderstanding or honest mistake:** this way, even if it was intentional, the other person has a graceful way out. If you back people into a corner, they will fight; it's not worth it.
- **Don't be passive–aggressive:** passive–aggressive behaviour is what happens when people are afraid of being angry, so they show their anger in a way that doesn't *look* angry. In the example above, if you had to work the weekend anyway, a passive–aggressive behaviour would be to call in sick. Gossiping about the person who did the off duty, getting even by scheduling them for 3 weeks of weekends when you do the off duty, getting revenge in sneaky ways – these are all passive–aggressive behaviours. Don't act that way.
- **Don't be manipulated:** people will react to confrontations in different ways, and they may act one way while really meaning

something else. 'Oh, sorry, I thought it was your weekend to work, I'll take care of it for next week, promise' could mean 'You caught me, but I'm not doing anything about it, and if I can get away with it this time I'll probably try it again ...' Although you should try to accept what they are doing and saying at face value, pay attention and be aware that there could be other factors at work. It would be OK to say 'I'm sure it was a mistake but it is not my weekend, and I don't feel I should have to work it.'

- **Focus on solutions, not on blame/shame:** have some solutions and alternatives in mind when you start the confrontation.
- **Tell how *you* are feeling:** start statements with 'I feel ...', 'I want ...' and 'I need ...', not 'You do ...' or 'You make me ...'. Don't put words in people's mouths. Don't say 'We all ...' or 'Everyone thinks ...'. If you are the one asserting yourself, then speak only for yourself, unless you are there as a member of a group and the group has agreed that you speak for the other members.
- **Stick to your limits:** don't let yourself be manipulated or bullied. If you are being fair and reasonable, don't be afraid to raise your concerns at a higher level.
- **Remember the emotional and intellectual level of the person you are speaking to:** you may need to make allowances for people who are very young, very old, who have just been through something very traumatic, or who have some difficulty that affects the way they relate to other people.

Asserting yourself can be difficult, especially if you have been raised in a culture where it is not right to complain or it is wrong to speak up to people in authority. It takes practice. Find someone who is good at being assertive and ask him or her to help you. As you become more confident and experienced, it will become easier and more natural for you to be assertive.

Assertiveness is a powerful leadership trait and developing it will be good for your grades, your career and your level of stress.

BOUNDARIES

Let's be completely clear on boundaries: bad boundaries will get you into trouble, so learn good boundaries as a student and keep them during your nursing career. Nurses care intimately for people and it is easy for boundaries to become blurred. You have an obligation – to yourself, to your patients and to your colleagues – to keep your boundaries clear.

What are good boundaries?

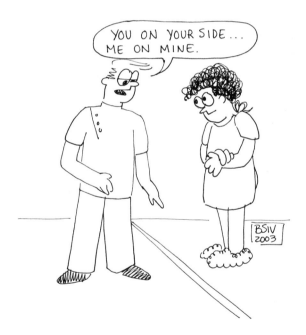

- Being attached enough to take care of someone but not so attached you want to take them home with you.
- Being able to say 'No' when it's appropriate.
- Being able to separate your personal life from who you are as a nurse (this is tough for many people).

Some patients will really get to you. You'll want to help them, support them and take care of them. But you have to remember your role and respect that there are things you can't do:

- Don't give patients your personal contact details.
- Don't do things that are inappropriate (buying alcohol, etc.).
- Never ever keep a 'secret'. What happens when the patient says 'Thanks for promising not to tell. I am going to kill myself tonight.'? If a patient ever says to you 'I'll tell you, but please don't tell anyone ...' say 'I might need to tell someone else, so if it's really something no one else can know, I'd feel better if you didn't tell me.' Don't ever promise to keep a secret: if you find out, once hearing the secret, that you must share it, it puts you in a terrible position. If a patient won't tell you because you won't promise not to tell, tell your mentor or more senior member of staff.
- Just because you are the nurse doesn't mean all the patient's problems are your problems. You are there to take care of the patient but you are one member of a team. If the patient has other problems – financial worries, relationship worries, etc. – don't let yourself be sucked into fixing things that you are neither trained nor equipped to cope with. Tell your mentor or another staff nurse what you know about the patient's problems.
- Don't tell too much about yourself. It's not appropriate to treat a patient like a friend – sharing information about your family and about your life outside work. It can also make it very difficult for patients to treat you like a nurse when they see you as a friend.

We can work so hard as nurses that we can forget that we don't have to be a nurse all the time. I remember letting it slip on one holiday that I was a nurse and I spent the rest of the week listening to people talk on and on about their constipation and their great-aunt's ear surgery!

You are probably very proud of being a nurse – and rightly so! But if you tell people you are a nurse, they may come to you and ask for help and advice. Or they might take advantage of your caring nature and bore you to death talking about things that no one else will listen to. They might even skip getting the help they really need and expect you to do things for them. As a student, you are not qualified to give advice and anyway, don't you have enough to do already? Remember the limitations of being a student and don't forget that if you don't take care of yourself, you won't be there to take care of anyone else.

At the beginning of this section I mentioned that bad boundaries are bad for your colleagues. Here's an example …

In America, I worked in a large team of community nurses. One day a nurse came in over an hour late for our meeting. She turned to the nurse on her left (I'll call her Sukie) and said angrily 'Look, you might think that doing Mrs King's shopping is OK when you do it, but then she expects me to do it!'

Sukie had a habit of being 'too good' to patients. Sukie did a little shopping, a little laundry, watered the plants… and that set up an expectation that we would all do the same. The patients didn't realize Sukie was doing 'extra'; they assumed it was part of the visiting nurse's role. Other nurses felt guilty when they said 'No' to patients Sukie said 'Yes' to and they were angry with Sukie as a result. Patients became angry when other nurses didn't do the same things that Sukie did.

Sukie was repeatedly passed over for promotion and struggled to get people to help her – they thought that if she had time to do extra then she had time to get her own work done. The situation was very unpleasant for everyone. And poor Sukie – all she was trying to do was help. She was an excellent nurse, very technically skilled; she just had very blurry boundaries. She didn't understand why everyone was so angry. She saw herself as a good nurse, felt isolated and was very hurt when she didn't get promoted.

The moral of the story? *Being 'too good' isn't too good.*

COMMUNICATION

There are three actual different types of communication:

- what you say or don't say and how you say (or don't say) it
- what your body language says
- what you write.

In this section, we are going to talk about how to communicate in a positive, non-threatening way; in Chapter 11, I will explain how to use good communication in your nurse's notes. Let me tell you a secret … sometimes, nurses don't really communicate well:

- We interrupt patients when they talk to us.
- We explain things instead of just accepting how patients feel.
- We make judgements.
- We switch discussion to things we can handle when we are stressed and when we feel defensive.
- We are busy; we focus on getting tasks done and see talking to patients as an interruption or a waste of time.
- We talk to our colleagues as though the patient isn't really there.

An example:

Mr Brown: 'Nurse, I'm really worried that I'm not getting any better.'

Nurse: 'Oh Mr Brown, you look great today …' (keeps putting linen away)

Mr Brown: 'Yes, OK …'(walks away)

What is Mr. Brown really trying to say? He's saying 'Nurse, I'm afraid – help me'. What is the nurse saying? 'Buzz off, I can't handle your problem right now – the linen is so much more important.' How would it be if it went this way?

Mr Brown: 'Nurse, I'm really worried that I'm not getting any better.'

Nurse: (stops what she is doing) 'Mr Brown, you have been unwell a long time and it must feel as though it's never going to get any better.' (leads patient to sit down to talk)

Mr Brown: 'Yes, I have been ill so long – am I dying and no one told me?'

Nurse: 'Mr Brown, I don't think you are dying but I can imagine it's very frustrating to be unwell for so long. Would you like me to ask the doctor to talk to you about how long it is taking to get better?'

Mr Brown: 'If it's not too much trouble …'

See the difference? In the second example, the nurse does something called 'reflecting'. Look at the first thing she says: the nurse took Mr. Brown's words and repeated them back to him. It shows that she was paying attention; it is a way of saying 'tell me more'.

Remember to make eye contact when you talk to people. Stop what you are doing. Move so that you are level with the other person. Therapeutic talking needs both people to be at the same physical level. You can't show how compassionate you are if you are towering over the other person.

It's not difficult to do… so why don't we all do it? Maybe we are very task oriented, and talking to the patient gets in the way of getting 'real' work done. Sometimes, patients and families talk about things that we can't fix and it's scary for us professional 'fixers', to be faced with not being able to do anything. Maybe we don't like people and we just don't want to be with them. In truth, sometimes we are genuinely busy and really don't have time.

So how can we be good communicators as nurses?

- **Be honest:** 'Mr Brown, I can't talk to you right now – can we have some time in a little bit so I can really pay attention?' (then make sure you *do* go back!).
- **Remember that you don't have to fix everything:** sometimes, patients just want to know that someone else understands how they feel.
- **Feelings and perceptions are personal, there is no right or wrong:** if a patient says 'You are ignoring me!' you don't need to argue with them even if you are sure you are not ignoring them. It's OK if patients' feelings are different than yours. You don't have to be 'right'. 'Mr Brown, I'm sorry that you feel I am ignoring you. How can I help you?'
- **A little sympathy goes a long way:** 'Mr Brown, I'm sorry that this is taking so long, you must be very tired of all this.' OK, it's not your fault but when *you* are frustrated doesn't it feel good to know that people understand?
- **Don't take it personally:** sometimes patients and families (or colleagues!) will act in ways that are very aggressive or

unpleasant. Try to be understanding and patient. This doesn't mean you should let yourself be abused, but try to see things from the other person's point of view. Someone they love is sick, perhaps in pain and, they are afraid. They are not at their best. Don't argue or wind people up. They aren't really angry with you – they are angry about their circumstances.

- **Smile, touch, laugh, cry, be yourself:** as long as you don't go overboard – and you remember your boundaries – it's usually OK to show your feelings, although you need to use good judgement. A friend once said 'You can always tell the best nurses – they are the ones who cry ...' What he meant was that nurses who show their feelings aren't cold or distant about the work they do. People who are ill want to be cared for by people, not machines. The real exception to this is when you are caring for people who have a mental illness or learning disability that could result in them misinterpreting your intentions. You don't want to give the wrong message.

- **Don't treat patients like they aren't there:** don't talk to your friend when you make Mr Brown's bed, talk to *him*. Don't chat to someone else when you are taking his observations, it will hurt his feelings. He's stuck in the hospital worried about getting better and he hears you chatting about your big night out – how do you think it makes him feel? Take opportunities to communicate. And what about Mrs Cecile, who has had a stroke and is unconscious? Talk to her too. Maybe, just maybe, she can hear you. You might be the only person who speaks to her all day.

- **Explain things when you do them:** how would you feel if you were in bed, couldn't see, couldn't talk, couldn't move and all of a sudden someone was washing your genitals? Try to put yourself in the patient's place. Ask permission, even if the person is unconscious. 'Mr Akram, I'd like to give you a bath, OK?' A small thing can make such a difference.

- **Be polite:** say 'please', 'thank you' and 'excuse me'. Address people by their surname (Mr, Mrs, Miss) until told otherwise.

Introduce yourself. Ask permission. Don't assume Mr Akram will allow you to call him Ronnie; ask him if you can.

- **Don't force a patient to interrupt your conversation with your colleague:** as soon as patients are near or approaching, make eye contact to let them know they have your full attention. Don't make them wait – you can talk to your friend anytime.
- **Talk is therapy just like medicine:** you don't need to be a professional counsellor to talk to patients. Just listen and be a friend (a friend with good boundaries!) Make sure, however, that you stay within the scope of your role.
- **Keep your body language open:** smile, make eye contact, don't tower over people when you speak to them, use touch when appropriate.
- **Speak plainly:** 'Mrs Gardner, despite the complication of peritonitis after your laparoscopic appendectomy, the registrar feels that your course of cephalothin is resolving this and your prognosis is improving.' Do you think Mrs Gardner understood that? Why not just say 'The antibiotics we are giving you are helping and you are getting better'. Don't call the patient's jaw a 'mandible', call it a 'jaw'. If you must use big words to impress your friends and family, fair enough, but always speak at the level you know the patient will understand. Make sure the patient and his or her family knows they can stop and ask you what something means. Don't ever tell a patient something that you don't understand the meaning of!

COPING WITH STRESS

Stress, what a wonderful thing! Stress causes physiological responses that quicken our reflexes, help us learn and adapt, and get us out of trouble. However, if stress lasts too long we find ourselves getting tired, worn out and depressed. Our physiological coping skills start to backfire. We get 'stressed out'.

People have many different ways of dealing with stress. Some are negative:

- drinking, taking drugs, smoking
- food (eating too much or too little)
- becoming depressed
- withdrawal and isolation
- spending money
- being grouchy, irritable and aggressive.

Some people cope with stress in very positive ways:

- looking for solutions to the problems causing them stress
- exercising at the gym, going for a walk, taking up Tai Chi
- taking a break or a holiday
- going for counselling
- going out with friends and having a good time.

You are facing a very stressful time, from many different angles:

- you are financially stressed
- you are in a stressful profession
- you will become sleep deprived
- you will be learning a lot in a short period of time
- you will be exposed to the pain and suffering of people around you
- you will be worried about passing your course
- your important relationships could suffer
- you will find yourself juggling all kinds of priorities
- you will feel like you don't have any time
- responsibilities like housework, ironing, etc. could all feel overwhelming
- you will probably be working extra hours on top of your course
- you could feel bullied or harassed.

Depressed yet?

If you are, cheer up. It's never as bad as you are worried it could be. The whole point is knowing what you are really up against. Let me give you an example …

My husband and I go on holiday in Greece. I love Greece – the sea, the food, the people, the history – it's wonderful. People in Greece have a very relaxed attitude about everything, and I find it very frustrating. When we go to Greece, and I get impatient because the waiter is busy talking to his friends and has been ignoring us for half an hour, or the bus is twenty minutes late, and I start clucking and carrying on, my (incredibly patient and sensible) husband says 'Don't you love being in the Mediterranean?'

What he is intentionally reminding me is: I knew it was going to be like this when I went there, I can't change it, and if I keep getting frustrated the only person who will suffer is me (well, and him). We both know that I'll get stressed when those things happen. So he helps me recognize when it is happening.

Now, we plan ahead to prevent the stress. We don't go to a restaurant when we are starving, we go an hour before we really think we will want to eat. If we are in a hurry, we take a taxi instead of the bus. We plan to cope with the stress and it helps us just enjoy our holiday.

You need to do the same with nursing:

- **Know what stresses you:** some people are stressed by lateness or by having a lot to do, or even by having to ask other people for help. Know what your pet peeves are and plan on how to work with them. Know how to prevent the stress from adding up.
- **Have time for yourself:** many people find that spending good time with friends and family helps with stress. Taking a break, even when you are really busy, can help you calm down and focus on what needs to be done. Don't work yourself into a rut; take a day when you are not thinking about nursing, uni, your assignments … you will go back refreshed and with a clear mind.
- **Don't get into a pattern of bad coping:** coping with the ways you cope can be worse than the stress! If you cope by eating, drinking or going out, try to be aware that at some point you could go overboard and that too much of anything – even a good thing – can be harmful. Caffeine, chocolate, exercise and alcohol are good things in moderation but could add to, rather than resolve, stress if used excessively.

- **Don't hide or procrastinate:** don't stuff the 'final demand for payment notice' under the sofa. Don't call-in sick because you can't face your mentor. Don't leave your assignment until the last minute because you feel you don't know what to do. All these put off stress momentarily but make more stress in the end.

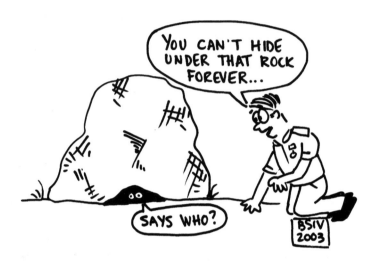

- **Accept that stress happens:** you *will* get stressed. Look at the context of that stress. Is it life threatening? Is it worth allowing yourself to get worked up about? Is anyone going to die? A dear friend once said 'The way I tell if I need to allow myself to get stressed over something is wondering if it would ever make the papers!'
- **Plan ahead for stress:** give yourself permission to not be perfect. When you are going into something that you know makes you stressed, look at yourself honestly and tell yourself it's OK. If it happens, it happens. Believe it or not, it will help you keep control.
- **Know who to go to for help:** if the stress really builds up, you could become depressed or have other physical problems. It's OK to seek help. Talk to your personal tutor, the student union advisor, your GP. If you start feeling as though you can't cope with anything, get help. It's normal to need help sometimes.

DELEGATION AND ORGANIZATION

These two concepts go hand in hand – delegation is sharing out your work with other people. Organization is how you organize your day and your workload to get everything done in a timely way. If you organize your work, you can see what things you need to delegate. Does that make sense?

Let's talk about delegating things first. You can't be everywhere and do everything as a nurse. One of the most difficult things for a student nurse to get used to is delegating tasks to other people. Yes, believe it or not, you will need to start delegating as soon as you start placements.

- You will need to prioritize; what can only be done by you and what can others do safely and appropriately?
- You will need to choose which tasks can wait until later and which must be done now.
- You will need to delegate to qualified nurses what you as a student do not feel safe or prepared for, or feel is not within your scope.

Think for a minute about life before your nursing course. Imagine you are with a partner and you have two children. You do the washing up, laundry, cooking, cleaning, shopping, ironing, mending, gardening – the list goes on.

Now, you have all these responsibilities plus you have the added responsibilities of your academic work and your placements. No one else can do your course so you know that you must always be the one to do the academic work, although you might ask someone else to get a book at the library for you or do something else that supports you.

Of the other tasks, you need to think, 'What can only I do?' You might decide that you must do the ironing and the shopping but that the other tasks can go to your partner and your children. You still help out when you can but you have certain responsibilities that come first. If an emergency should happen – one of your children is ill for example – you can rearrange a bit, but there are always certain things that only you can do.

The same is true in nursing. There will be some things that only you as a nurse can do, some things you can always pass off to someone else and some things in the middle that you may need to do or you might be able to delegate.

How do you decide what to delegate? Think of the following:

- Legally, can only a qualified nurse do this?
- According to trust policy, should only a qualified nurse do this?
- Does this task require a nursing judgement or skilled intervention?
- If I delegate it, does someone else have the appropriate training and knowledge to do it?
- If it is delegated, how badly could things go if it went wrong?
- Is there appropriate supervision and support for the person to whom I delegate this task?
- Am I skiving by asking someone else to do it?
- Is there anything to make me think it should not be delegated?
- What is the best use of my time, for my patient's best interest?

The answers to these questions will help you decide what you can delegate and what you should do yourself.

Delegating isn't easy, but you will need to do it. It's especially hard as a student but being able to delegate will show that you are thinking and behaving like a nurse.

When you delegate, you don't need to act like a general, ordering people about. You can simply ask someone to help you. Be polite, but know what you really want. When you ask someone to help you, you need to remember:

- What specifically do I want the other person to do, and when does it need to be done by?
- Do I want the other person to come back and tell me when it is done?
- Do I need to give the other person any additional information about what I need done?

Be specific. 'Sara, can you please get Mrs Jones and Mr Bradley ready to go home? I'd like it done as soon as you have a chance, they need to be ready to go by 11.30' is better than 'Sara, get the patients washed up!'

Don't just send someone off to do something for you because you are too lazy to do it yourself! If you wind up with extra time, then go and help out other people. Then, *they* will help *you* when *you* are running late.

Delegating starts with knowing what you have ahead of you for the day. In handover, make a note of all the things that have to be accomplished. Organizing your day starts here.

Now think about a typical handover. You have eight patients; you have two HCAs working with you, although one of them is going home at 11.00 a.m; it is now 8.00 a.m and you have the following things to accomplish for your eight patients:

- bed baths and bed making
- observations to be recorded
- medication rounds at 9.00 a.m.
- three dressings
- a preoperative assessment
- two patients are being discharged before lunch
- something to be picked up from the pharmacy for one of the patients being discharged.

Which things can only you do? What things could someone else do safely without you? Do some things have to be done before others? Make a 'to do' list and prioritize the items in order of their importance – put what must be done first at the top of the list. Star the things that only you can do.

This is where you need to start thinking about organization. If you look at the things ahead of you at the start of your shift, you will be able to plan your day.

Organization starts in handover. Prepare for handover by writing down the names and bed numbers of the patients before you go into handover. Use a three- or four-colour pen and when things

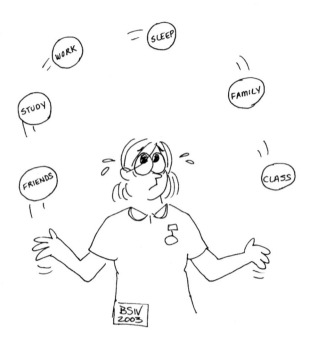

must be done, write them or circle them in another colour. Then you can see them easily and cross them off as they are done. Make your to do list, triage and decide what needs to be done first, and then go out and get your work done – think about which things need to be done first, and do them first! Try to plan your work in a way that is considerate to other people. For example, if you wait to do the preoperative assessment until theatre calls for the patient, then someone is going to have to wait while you do it. If you do it right away, then the patient is already prepared and no one has to wait. Time management skills are absolutely essential. As a student and as a nurse you will always feel like you're juggling a lot of balls in the air at one time.

To be organized, you need to remember the following:

- What things are likely to interrupt me, and how can I plan ahead for them?
- What things can wait until later?

- What things can I do to make things better for the next shift?
- What things are best done by someone else?

Think about the preoperative assessment in the list of things to accomplish above. You know that sometime during the morning you will be interrupted by a phone call from theatre. If the patient is ready, that call will last 1 minute; if the patient isn't ready, you will have to explain and tell theatre when the patient will be ready and, when you go to do the assessment, it will be more stressful because you are in a hurry. Doing the assessment first thing would save you phone time, an interruption and a lot of stress.

All during your work day new things will pop up and demand a place on your to do list. If you always know which things can wait, you know where you can put new problems on the list. One way to know what things can wait is to 'triage' things on your list. Triage means sorting things out according to how urgent they are. I use an 'ABCD' system:

A   Absolutely must get done before other things.
B   Better get done sooner rather than later.
C   Can wait until later.
D   Don't worry about it.

Absolutely must get done ...

These are the things, like getting the patient ready for theatre, that must be done before I can really concentrate on doing other things; things that if I don't do them now, someone is going to interrupt me to do them while I am doing something else. Things other people may be waiting for before they can carry on: for me to find an X-ray, to give pain medication, etc.

Better get done sooner ...

These are the things that although not life or death, are important and need to be done. Although no one will die if I leave them in bed an extra half an hour, it is unpleasant to be left stuck in bed so I must get people up, washed and dressed after I have done all the things that can't wait. Sometimes you have to do some 'Better get done's ...' while waiting for opportunities to get 'Absolutely ...' tasks finished, for example, if you need a urine sample before a person goes to theatre (an 'Absolutely ...') take the time to get the person to the loo and get them washed up at the same time.

Can wait ...

These are the 'when you have a chance' things. Things like going to the pharmacy to get something not needed until the afternoon. Some paperwork and administrative tasks are 'Can waits'. You just have to make sure they get done.

Don't worry ...

Some things are nice to do but if you don't get them done it won't affect your patient care. Things like tidying up the break room, putting together documents in advance for new admissions.

Sometimes things will go up in rank: I had changing Mr Long's bed down as a 'Can wait ...', until his IV came out and blood went all over the bed, at which point it became an 'Absolutely ...'.

Some things will go down in rank: it was imperative that I give Mr Sullivan his prep. for endoscopy before 10.00 a.m., until they cancelled the procedure!

When I make a to-do list, I rank things according to my ABCD list. I don't really worry about Bs until all the As are done. I just keep going. I try not to take a break or get distracted until I have at least most, if not all, the 'Absolutely ...' tasks done. Although it isn't always realistic to do things that way, I try. If someone throws a new task my way, I rank it and it gets its place in my priorities. If I have a chance to get something else done easily while doing one task, I try to fit it in.

It takes time and practice to get used to organizing your work for a shift. Watch the way others do it. How does it feel to work with someone who isn't very organized? How does it feel when someone helps the shift go by smoothly? If you find someone who always seems to have things under control, ask how they organize themselves and learn from them.

ETHICS

Nurses work within a number of different ethical frameworks. Your university will let you know which specific model it will use during the ethics and law module you will take. Basically, ethics boils down into three main issues:

- do no harm/do good (non-maleficence/beneficence)
- trustworthiness/truth-telling and honesty/justice and fairness
- respect for personhood/respect for individual autonomy.

In some ethical models, these will be teased out into more categories, but I have found it easier to think about them trimmed down to just these three.

Do no harm/do good (non-maleficence/ beneficence)

The first cardinal rule of nursing, and of medicine, is '*Do no harm*'. As a nurse, you must look at the way your actions affect your patient. You must always consider: are my actions causing harm? What is the benefit for my patient? The patients and their families should never be worse off for knowing you! This doesn't mean that you won't, as a nurse, do things that cause discomfort, because we all know that it's inevitable that we will. It doesn't mean you won't do things that the patient doesn't like to have done. The key is that everything you do must ultimately be in the patient's best interest and not make anything any worse for them. '*Doing no harm*' also means that you need to keep good boundaries and stay within the limitations and scope of your role as a student (and eventually as a nurse).

Trustworthiness/truth-telling and honesty/ justice and fairness

Nursing is one of the most trusted professions in the world. Just because you are a nurse (or even a nursing student) people are going to make assumptions about you and your character. They are going to assume that you are a good and honest person. It's important for people to feel that the people taking care of them and their families are people who they can trust. You have an obligation to uphold that trustworthiness. Part of the way you prove you are trustworthy is by being honest. The catch is, as a nurse, telling the truth isn't always as simple as just blurting out the most truthful answer you can think of. You have to find a way to tell the truth that *does no harm*. Don't ever lie to a patient. It's better to say 'I don't know' or 'I need to ask someone else to discuss this with you'. You also prove your trustworthiness by following the legal and professional codes for your practice, and behaving in a fair and just way.

Respect for personhood/respect for individual autonomy

As a nurse, you have an obligation to put aside any personal biases or prejudices. You have to see each of your patients and their families as people who are deserving of the best care you can offer.

You must always remember that patients have the right to make decisions for themselves, even when those decisions are not the ones we as nurses or medical people would make for them. Some people may not have the capacity to make decisions for themselves: it is your obligation to do the best you can to make the decisions you believe in your heart would be the ones these patients would make for themselves if they were able to. Sometimes, we put a lot of pressure on people to make the decision we want them to make. To a limited extent, we can use our influence as carers to manipulate patients into doing what we think is best. But remember, there is a difference between someone saying, 'Nurse, I don't want to do this ...' and a person saying, 'No, I will *not* do this'. There is a difference between getting someone up when they have just had an operation and would rather stay in bed and giving someone a medication or treatment that they don't want. Use your communication skills, educate your patients and really listen to them. Even patients who have diminished capacity to make decisions – the elderly infirm, the mentally ill, the learning disabled, someone with an altered level of consciousness, children – still have the right to be treated with respect, dignity and with a regard for their personal beliefs, wishes and views. It's not always easy.

Ethics is not a clear-cut process. There is no easy way to make sure you are making the most ethical decision. There is no single ethical principle that is greater than, or more important than, the others. There are some ways you can work towards making ethically correct decisions:

- **Know yourself:** do you have any prejudices, biases or strong beliefs that could cause conflict with your patients? For example, are you afraid of people of a different colour? Do you have strong religious beliefs that could make you feel that another religion is 'wrong' or 'bad'? Do you have strong pro-life or pro-choice beliefs? Could you take care of a prisoner who was convicted of rape or child molestation? It's OK to have strong beliefs. You just can't inflict your views on patients or their families and carers. You must be aware of those strong feelings that could cause conflict and develop self-awareness about how to prevent them from surfacing when you are working as a nurse. If you ever find yourself caring for someone and you can't get past feelings that are making you struggle to see the patient as a person worthy of respect, then let someone know and remove yourself from caring for that person. *Do no harm.*

- **Be a reflective practitioner:** reflect on your experiences, look for the ethics in your decisions and actions. When you are making a decision, consciously look for the ethical elements and reflect later on what you needed to think about.
- **Try to see yourself and your actions from the patient's perspective:** seeing yourself and your actions from outside yourself is essential for growth. It is a key element in critical thinking. When you see things you aren't comfortable with, make a plan for changing them. Don't worry about not being perfect – just look for places where you can learn and grow as a person and as a nurse.
- **Develop your own philosophy about nursing:** if you have your own philosophy about nursing, about yourself as a nurse and about the type of nursing you would like to do, it will be easier for you to make decisions. Yes, I am talking about actually sitting down and writing out a philosophy. Starting with 'I believe that nursing is …' and 'I believe that as a nurse I …'. Review your philosophy every so often. Carry it with you and, when you are frustrated, stressed or struggling to make a difficult decision, re-read it. If you outgrow your philosophy, update it. It will help keep you centred. It doesn't need to be an A4 page – just a couple of lines.
- **Ask someone else for help:** it's perfectly acceptable to go to a trusted colleague, teacher or mentor and say, 'I'm struggling with this …'. When you are faced with difficult or confusing situations, talk about them. You should never have to make decisions in isolation.
- **Be an advocate:** if you find yourself in a situation where someone has blatantly behaved in a way that you feel is unethical, it is your obligation to speak up. Always do the best you can to be an advocate for your patients and their rights. Refuse to do anything that you feel that you ethically cannot do but support patients in making the decisions that they honestly believe are best for them. For example …

A man is brought into the A&E haemorrhaging from trauma. He tells you that he is a Jehovah's Witness and does not believe it is right to receive blood. He understands the consequences of his decision. You know that without blood he will probably die. You disagree with him but you respect his decision. You don't give him blood. If someone else decides to give blood anyway, you have to decide if you are going to challenge their actions or not. It's not easy, no matter what you decide. If you were the patient, what would you want someone to do for you?

You will be asked to make some very difficult decisions as a nurse. You will be there when people receive difficult and painful news. You will be there when people are struggling to make incredibly difficult decisions. You must always remember that, as a nurse, you must put your personal beliefs and feelings aside so that you can be the nurse the patient needs you to be. It can be incredibly difficult to do.

Let me give you an example …

I used to work on an ambulance. In a case I was called to, a young man who had been drinking had put his infant daughter in the car but not in an appropriate car seat. He fell asleep at the wheel, crashed the car and his daughter was very seriously injured. He was unhurt except for some cuts and bruises. The smell of alcohol was incredibly strong and I am sure every person there – fire fighters, police, paramedics – felt certain that the man was to blame for his daughter's injuries. Despite being angry with him, we still had to treat him with respect and compassion. It was incredibly hard for us – it's a normal thing to feel protective and worried about a small child – but we all had to remember that behaving in any but the most professional way would be wrong. He had done enough harm to himself without us making it worse. All right, there wasn't a lot of small talk going on; but we took good care of him and comforted him the best we could. We put being good carers ahead of being judgemental. After we dropped him off at the hospital we vented our frustration and anger about the situation to each other: he never saw anything from us but caring and compassion. (The little girl recovered completely.)

It takes reflection, self-awareness and thoughtfulness to be a good nurse. Knowing and understanding ethics is a giant step towards this goal.

There may be times you will be called upon to justify your decisions as being ethically correct. If you can show that you have self-awareness, that you understand the ethical principles and that you put thought and consideration into the decisions you make, you will be able to trust that the decisions you make are good ones.

LEADERSHIP

Some students (and, sadly, some nurses) believe that a student nurse cannot be a leader. Many of the things we have discussed in this chapter are important parts of leadership. Leadership is about being the kind of person other people can rely upon and can look up to. It's about making good decisions and being a good role model.

Many people think leadership is about being charismatic and having other people like and admire them. It can happen that way but there is something much more important at stake than personal power and importance. Good leaders improve the NHS as a whole and, as a result, improve the care we give. Even just one student nurse can improve the NHS. Surprised? If you as a student make a conscious decision to make things better, you *can* do it. How?

- Keep your practice based in evidence.
- Wash your hands and challenge other people to wash theirs.
- Challenge bad practice.
- Be self-aware.
- Don't fall into the 'It's not the right way but it's the way we do it here' trap.
- Always try to see things from the patient's perspective.

These things might not seem like leadership activities, but they are. It will help to understand why if you understand norms. Norms are the values held by a group of people. They aren't written rules but the 'way we do things'. The pressure that makes us obey norms is the approval or disapproval of other people.

Norms

Let's apply this to clinical practice …

Imagine that in a particular hospital all the day shifts start at 7.00 a.m. On ward C2, everyone is very particular about being on time. The manager, the sisters – everyone is always there, and ready to work, at 7.00 a.m. sharp. You make a conscious effort to be there at 7.00 a.m. too, because you know that everyone else does.

When you go to ward Z2, things aren't so strict. The ward manager gets there at 7:20 a.m., handover starts at 7:20 a.m. and nurses are still getting there at 7:10 and 7:15 a.m. How long do you think it would take before you started being late, too?

That's a norm. Although the rule says 'Be here at 7.00 a.m.', the norm says 'We will not make a fuss if you are late'.

Now, imagine again that the ward manager from C2 takes over for the ward manager of Z2. She shows up on time. She says something to nurses who are late. People start showing up on time.

The manager's disapproval caused people to start to follow the rule again. If the manager isn't there for 3 weeks it could slip back into the old norm – unless leaders amongst the staff keep the new 'on time' norm going. Eventually, the new norm will stick and people will adhere to it even if the manager isn't there.

That's where you, as a student, can be a leader. If you know the right way to do things, and you make sure you do the best you can to do things the right way, you are helping good norms to survive.

One point to remember: think about what we discussed in the 'communication' part of this chapter. Try to make your point about good practice without stabbing people with that point! You will need to use tact and diplomacy, 'Oi, what's wrong with you, we don't do it that way!!!' is not the way to promote good practice! The way you say something is important.

If you work in an area that has hoists but still uses lifting to move people, you are a leader when you say, 'I am not prepared to lift; I'll go and get the hoist'. You are encouraging other people to do the right thing. Just criticizing someone for not using the hoist isn't the right way.

Can you imagine the decrease in infections if everyone washed their hands properly? You as a student could be a leader – simply by making sure you wash your hands properly. Other people see you do it and it encourages and reminds them. You know how difficult it can be to do something when you don't see anyone else doing it – start a positive trend! That's leadership.

You can be a leader in another way, too. You can get involved in student advocacy, through your union, the student union, or as a student rep for your group. It's not easy and it can be stressful but often there are opportunities to learn about leadership, genuinely help other people – and to build up your CV.

Concerns about good leadership go from students to the very highest levels of nurses. Not long ago, I was in a meeting with some very high-level nurses and we discussed leadership, management and governance.

Governance

Governance is a very important issue for nurses: it's the way we make sure that the right things are being done by the right people. You will hear about clinical governance, which is how we make absolutely sure the NHS is prepared and able to give the best, most appropriate care to the people who need that care.

According to the Chief Medical Officer, Sir Liam Donaldson, clinical governance is:

> A system through which NHS organizations are accountable for continuously improving the quality of their services and safeguarding high standards of care, by creating an environment in which clinical excellence will flourish.

Sir Liam Donaldson also said:

> Above all, though, clinical governance is about the culture of NHS organisations. A culture where openness and participation are encouraged, where education and research are properly valued, where people learn from failures and blame is the exception rather than the rule, and where good practice and new approaches are freely shared and willingly received.

Put simply, management is about making good decisions about resources, about human relations, and about following the guidelines and policies properly. It's running the business side of things. Anyway, the management consultant in this meeting told us, 'Leadership is where governance and management overlap.' What he meant was:

- Leadership is about taking risks, but those risks have to be taken with an awareness of policy, evidence and people's needs.
- Leadership isn't management but it considers the needs of managers.
- Leadership improves care and supports people in improving their ability to improve care (governance).

The *NHS Plan* (DoH 2000) clearly states that leadership is required at all levels. It doesn't say 'except students'. So, how can you be a leader?

- Be politically well informed: know the trust, local and national policies, and the national initiatives, that relate to your area of nursing.
- Know theory as well as practice, and relate the two.
- Promote and role-model good practice (support good norms).
- Challenge other people (with respect, of course) to follow good practice.
- Don't let your standards slide.
- Look for opportunities to improve things. My mentor Fiona Malem told me 'Don't step over something – stop and fix it.' The person who finds the problem is the one who must take responsibility for it.
- Know the tools of your trade: assertiveness, coping with stress, good communication, delegation, time management and organization and ethics are important, along with your clinical skills and knowledge.
- Respect other people – colleagues, patients, families, carers, other professionals – for their abilities and contributions.

There's a lot more to leadership than this but this is a good foundation. Don't start out in leadership trying to change the world – just make sure you do the best *you* personally can. You may be surprised and find that other people start to follow you – and that's the way leaders are made.

One last note: if you think that being a leader means being powerful, you are right. There is a lot of power in having the approval of other people. If you are going into nursing because you like having power, well, put this book down and start looking for a different career. Still here? Oh good! Just remember, power doesn't make you any *better* than anyone else. Having more power just means having the responsibility to use that power and influence wisely. Remember the links between governance, management and leadership. There are negative leaders – the gossips, the people who become caught up in traditional roles and power, the people who resist change even when evidence shows that change is needed. Standing up to these kinds of leaders is very intimidating but it can be done simply by refusing to follow them.

As nurses, we are all equals with the same obligation to give the best care we are able to give at our level of education and experience. I don't know where the quote is from, but I have this written in the front of my diary:

> ❝ Those whom the gods would bring to their knees they first make proud. ❞

It was a reminder to myself, when I became a national-level advocate as a nursing student, that I would be useless if I didn't keep things in perspective. That's another key element in leadership: just be yourself.

When you see good leaders, you will know them. They are the people who inspire you, who give you confidence and who role-model the kind of nurse you want to be. Watch them and learn from them: that's the best way to learn leadership. And as you learn to be a leader, other people will be learning from you.

REFERENCES

Department of Health 2000 The NHS plan. HMSO, London
You can find out more about clinical governance from the Department of Health website: www.doh.gov.uk/clinical governance

7

Cracking the Code

6 When I started, I felt like I would never understand what everyone was talking about. It made me feel so stupid! Now, I'm in my third year and I can usually figure out words on my own ... 9

Final year nursing student

INTRODUCTION TO THE LANGUAGE OF NURSES

Medical people speak a special language full of large words and strange abbreviations. We seem to love the jargon and tongue-twisting words. Why?

- they are part of the tradition of nursing and medicine
- it's like shorthand where you can say something in one word that would take ten to explain normally
- it sets us apart from 'non-medical' people. It's like being in a special club with a secret code!

If a person told you that your patient was having a cabbage, what would you think? To a qualified nurse, a cabbage (CABG) is a type of heart surgery! A nurse talking to another nurse will use CABG instead of saying 'coronary artery bypass graft'.

A quick story … I was caring for a patient on a morning shift, and she was having heart bypass surgery (a CABG) that afternoon. From midnight the night before, she had been NBM (nothing by mouth) so she would have an empty stomach when she went to theatre (it reduces the risk of vomiting when under anaesthesia). I went to talk to her, asking how she felt. She said she was hungry but didn't mind because she was having cabbage that afternoon and she loved cabbage! The SHO (senior house officer) had told her she was having her CABG that afternoon, and she misunderstood.

Moral of the story? Speak 'nurse-ese' to your colleagues, but plain English to your patients.

NURSING/MEDICAL JARGON

You will encounter a whole new world of words and meanings when you start your nursing course. Everyone who has been around for a while will use them, and will probably forget that you might not have a clue what they are talking about. If you have been an HCA or worked in healthcare before, you are a step ahead. But whether you have been an HCA or are brand new to nursing, don't be afraid to ask what words and terms mean.

Here is a very brief list of new things you will be hearing about …

Word/ phrase	Meaning
Bottle	A urinal, a bottle that men can pee in when they can't go to the loo
Bank (or agency) staff	Nurses working for an outside organization that places them in different areas to meet staffing needs
Bed rest	The patient should stay in bed. He or she might be able to get up to the bed side to use a commode: you need to ask. 'Strict bed rest' means the patient must stay in bed at all times
Bowl	A basin that a person can wash in
Clinical waste/ yellow bags	Things that are yellow (such as bin bags) usually contain items soiled with blood or body fluids, or that have been used in patient care. This is clinical waste. Clinical waste is disposed of in a special way

(continued)

Word/ phrase	Meaning
Commode chair	A chair with wheels, that has a bed pan in it
D grade	A D-grade nurse is a basic staff nurse. E-grade nurses are more senior, F grade is a sister, G grade is a sister/team leader, H is a manager. A and B grades are often health care assistant grades. These gradings are being replaced by Agenda for Change (see Appendix 6)
Domestics	The people who clean, often serve tea, etc. (good friends to have!)
Handover	When the present shift tells the new shift about the patients and what they need
HCA/nurse auxiliary	A person who works helping nurses and delivering care at a certain level under supervision of a nurse. Different places use different titles
HO/SHO	House officer (HO)/senior house officer (SHO) – medical students and newly qualified doctors go through a progression of titles and jobs while they are being prepared for practice. House officers are newly graduated, senior house officers have been around a while. They are organized into teams under consultants
Kidney basin	A kidney-shaped bowl
NBM	Nil by mouth or nothing by mouth – the patient can't eat or drink anything at all
Off duty	The time schedule. There are different shifts: 'earlies', 'lates', 'nights' and 'twilights' … there may be others. Ask the staff what times shifts start and end
Porters	Transport people who transport patients to their appointments, tests, etc. and who also bring mail, supplies, etc. to areas
Sectioned	When a person is 'sectioned', they can be held in the hospital against their will
Sharps	Pointy things: needles, but also clinically contaminated items that could poke through a bin bag (glass tubes, etc.). These go into a sharps container
Sister	A senior nurse. Male 'sisters' are called charge nurses
Sluice	The ward's 'dirty room'. Usually where you find bedpans, wash basins, soap, commodes, bins, a place to flush away body fluids, etc.
TTOs	To take out – medications that patients take home with them

This list is not complete by any means but I hope it will give you a bit of a head start.

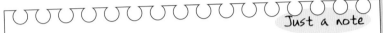

Just a note

Don't be ashamed of being new. If you really don't know what something means, ask. Don't just hope that no one will notice. Someone will! Yes, people might tease you a bit if you ask about something, but at least you are learning and anyone who criticizes you for learning isn't worth worrying about.

MEDICAL TERMINOLOGY IN GENERAL

Knowing some basics will help you to decipher medical terms. It is helpful to know that words in medicine are usually based on Latin or Greek words. There are three basic parts to most medical words: the prefix, the root, and the suffix. Here's an example …

'Electrocardiogram'. For now, just try to identify the different sections.

In electrocardiogram, you can see three main parts: 'electro', 'cardio' and 'gram'.

- 'electro' means electrical
- 'cardio' means pertaining to the heart
- 'gram' means a measurement or test.

Put the meanings of the smaller words together, and you have 'An electrical test of the heart'.

If you understand basic roots, prefixes and suffixes, you will have a clue to what the bigger words mean. Understanding the medical words for the different parts of the body, and the way their arrangement is described, can help you understand anatomy and different procedures, tests and medical problems. It will make it easier for you to understand what is being said in reports and in notes, to help you communicate clearly with other professionals, and help you explain things for your patients and their families.

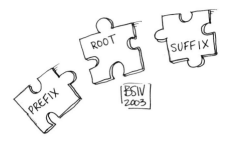

ANATOMICAL POSITIONS AND DESCRIPTIONS

There is a position known as the 'anatomical position'. Every description of the arrangement of the body is based on this position. Imagine someone facing you, standing on their tiptoes, and their arms by the sides with palms facing you. This is the 'anatomical position'.

Everything you can see from the front is 'anterior'. Everything you would need to look at from the back is 'posterior' or 'dorsal'. So, when you 'sit on your posterior', it quite literally means your back side!

Now, imagine a line cutting the person right in half, from the top of the head, the middle of the face, right through the centre of the body. That is the midline. Things close to the midline are 'medial', things away from the midline are 'lateral'.

'Superior' means top, or above, and 'inferior' means below or under. But the next terms are a bit more difficult:

- 'abduction', means to take away from the midline of the body (abduct means to take away)
- 'adduction' means to bring in towards the midline (to add it to the body)
- 'proximal' means closer
- 'distal' means further away
- 'flexion' is to bend a joint
- 'extension' is to stretch the joint out again
- 'transverse' means to go across

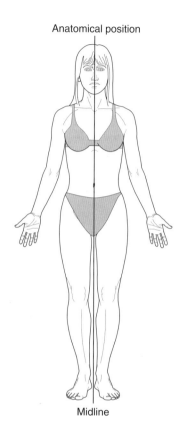

Anatomical position

Midline

- 'ascending' means to go up, 'descending' means to go down
- superior means above, inferior means below.

These terms are used in descriptions, for example:

- 'The skin graft was taken from the posterior forearm' (the graft was taken from the back of her arm).
- 'She had a large medial laceration on her ankle' (the inside of her ankle had a large cut).

They are also used in the names of different parts of the body:

- transverse colon
- medial meniscus
- adductor tendon.

It's always better when you can to say 'the top one was 2 × 2 centimetres' instead of using big bulky words, but many other professionals will use the big words. Don't use them if you aren't comfortable with them, but you should at least know what they mean. So, try the following:

1.   Which is more distal to the shoulder, the fingers or the elbow?
2.   Which is medial (in the anatomical position), the little finger or the thumb?
3.   If you drew a line across your belly, from hip to hip, would that line be transverse, ascending or descending?
4.   When you lift your knee to go up a step, is it extension or flexion?

The answers …

1.   The fingers, because they are further away from the shoulder, away from the centre of the body.
2.   The little finger, because it is closer to the centre or midline of the body.
3.   Transverse, because it goes across.
4.   Flexion, because you are bending your knee.

WORD ROOT BASICS

Now, time to learn about roots, prefixes and suffixes. Try to see these as pieces of a puzzle, which when put together in the right order will give you the whole picture.

Root words are the basic words taken from (usually) either Latin or Greek. A list of the most common ones appears in Appendix 7. Some things will have more than one root word referring to them, like the kidneys, which can be referred to using the roots 'renal' or 'nephr'. It takes time to get used to them but once you get used to hearing them they will make sense. After you have a root, you can use a suffix and/or a prefix to change the meaning.

COMMON SUFFIXES AND PREFIXES

Suffixes and prefixes are modifiers. Usually, the prefix modifies the root word and the suffix tells you something about the prefix and the root word. Here's an example …

Anuria. 'A' means 'no' or 'absent'; 'uri' means 'urine'; and an 'a' at the end means ' a condition'. So 'anuria' means that the patient is not putting out any urine, for some reason.

Try another one …

Cholecystitis. 'Chole' means gall; 'cyst' is a bladder, so you know that the 'chole' part (the prefix), is telling you which bladder we are talking about; 'itis' at the end of a word means an inflammation. This word is telling you the person has an inflamed gall bladder. If it were just cystitis, that would mean an inflammation of the urinary bladder.

One more: if 'chole' means gall, and 'lith' means stone, what is a cholelith? It's a gall stone!

Appendix 7 contains a list of root words, prefixes and suffixes. Some words won't follow the rules but most will. Soon, you will be amazing your friends and family with your difficult-to-pronounce new vocabulary. But remember, if you as a student nurse had to struggle to understand it, so will your patients. Speak in fancy medical talk to colleagues but speak plainly and clearly when explaining things to patients and families. They won't be impressed by big words: they'll just be intimidated.

8

Drug Calculations and Medication Administration

> ❝ I was on a bank shift, doing the drug rounds in a large nursing home. None of the patients wore identification bracelets – they all had their pictures in the drug book. As I went to give one patient a handful of pills I checked her against her photo. Slight lady, blue hair, big glasses ... I looked in her slippers and cardigan, and they had my patient's name. I asked her if her name was Lily and she said yes. Right picture, right room, right name – right patient. As I handed her the pills, she said, 'I haven't seen the blue ones before, and there are so many! I usually only get one.' An alarm went off in my head. I hit the pills out of her hand just as she was about to put them in her mouth. I got a nurse auxiliary who worked there full time to identify the patient – it wasn't Lily, it was another tiny, blue-haired old lady with thick glasses and a penchant for wandering and wearing other people's clothes. The medications I was giving her could have killed her. In all my years of nursing, I have never forgotten this, and it still makes cold chills go down my spine. ❞

Experienced nurse

In this chapter

Giving medication is only a small part of nursing but it can be dangerous. Having good skills and awareness will protect your patients – and your career as a student and as a nurse.

Although in this chapter I will do the best I can to give you a handy reference to jog your memory, you need to practise and become comfortable with conversions and calculations. I strongly suggest you get a book like *Nursing Calculations* by John Gatford and Nicole Phillips – it covers all the basics and will give you valuable practice.

BASIC CONVERSION OF UNITS

Basic numeracy is essential for nurses. If you are unclear about basic maths, your university should provide you with support to become more adept at the basics. If you know you have serious problems with basic calculations, ask your personal tutor, your library/learning resource centre or the student union about special courses to help you. Even if you are OK on the basics, keep a calculator handy and double-check your calculations with another nurse.

Basic measurements

Name of unit	Symbol	What it measures
Metre	m	Length
Gram	gm or g	Mass
Litre	L	Fluid

Getting used to the metric system in nursing can be challenging. The best way to get used to it is to practice. You will find other units of measure:

1000 units	Unit	1/100 units	1/1000 units	1/1 000 000 units
Kilometre	Metre (m)	Centimetre (cm)	Millimetre (mm)	
Kilolitre	Litre (L)	Centilitre (cL)	Millilitre (mL)	
Kilogram	Gram (g)	Centigram	Milligram (mg)	Microgram (mcg or μg)

Abbreviations are useful but you should only abbreviate when it will be absolutely clear what you mean. And make sure you use good, clear handwriting. Print! Think what could happen if someone misunderstood you.

This book can't teach you all about conversions but there is one small trick that will help you ... a way to remember which way the decimal point moves in metric conversions. If you don't know how to convert in the metric system, it can be very confusing. This might help:

- To convert from a larger unit to a smaller one, the decimal point moves to the right.
- To convert from a smaller unit to a larger one, the decimal point moves left.
- You move the decimal point a number of places based on the difference between the units. It's usually three places.

Example: you know that a kilogram contains 1000 milligrams (1 kg = 1000 mg). The difference between these two units, in 0s, is three places. So, you would move the decimal three places to the right to change kilograms into milligrams. If you have 250 kilograms (250.000 kilograms), you have 250 000 milligrams. If you had 250 milligrams, you would have 0.000250 kilograms).

It's very simple once you get used to it. You'll just need to practice. You also need to get comfortable with changing between metric and imperial measurements:

- 1 inch = 2.54 centimetres
- 1 kilogram = 2.2 pounds
- 1 stone = 14 pounds = 6.37 kilograms

This section has only the most basic units listed: as you find others, write them down inside the back cover of this book. You will remember them more easily if you write them down yourself.

It takes practice to get conversions right and you won't be alone if you feel a little confused about them. You will get used to it, and soon you will be an expert. Honest!

Summary

- You shouldn't abbreviate when writing units like milligrams and micrograms.
- You need to know how to convert units from the metric system into imperial measurements, and back again.
- You need reliable basic maths skills.

FORMULA FOR DRUG CALCULATIONS

Calculations will be based on one of the units of measurement. The most common error is in converting one unit of measure to another.

Sometimes a medication must be titrated (calculated based on an individual) to body weight or to body surface area (for example, a patient will receive 1 mg/kg of body weight). You always need to do the calculations using the same unit of measurement. This means there will be times you have to convert between units. If you are unsure of your conversions, have someone else double-check. It is good practice for any nurse to have someone double-check a calculation anyway!

Children's nurses will use special types of formulae and calculations. Children are not miniature adults; they are patients with very specific needs. Please get your information for these kinds of calculations from your mentor and from paediatric/children's nursing texts. I haven't put them here because I don't want you to take anything for granted when using them. The basics will still apply, but there are some very specific and important considerations you have to keep in mind; things too detailed for me to go into here.

In summary:

- drug calculations can take many different forms
- you can't calculate a dosage until everything uses the same unit of measure

- the most likely place you will make a mistake is in converting from one unit of measure to another
- you should always have another nurse double-check your calculations.

The most basic calculation is:

Dose = (dose needed/dose on hand) × dose unit

Try this out ...

You have 250-milligram capsules (so your dose unit is a 250 mg capsule) and you need to give 750 milligrams.

Dose = (750 mg/250 mg) × one 250 mg capsule

Dose = three 250 mg capsules

You need to make sure you have the same unit of measurement or this formula won't work. The same formula works for other types of units. Try liquid ...

You have heparin 1000 units in 5 mL. You need 5000 units. How much heparin do you give?

Dose = (5000 units/1000 units) × 5 mL

Dose = (5) × 5 mL

Dose = 25 mL

What if it was the other way around ...

You have 5000 units in 5 mL, but only need 1000 units?

Dose = (1000 units/5000 units) × 5 mL

Dose = (1/5) × 5 mL

Dose = 1 mL

What a useful formula this is! There are others but personally I find that having just one and being good at it is what is best.

SAFE AND RESPONSIBLE ADMINISTRATION OF MEDICATION

So, now you know you have the right amount of the medication you want to give. Think back to the quote at the beginning of the chapter – there is more to medication administration than getting the dose right:

> The administration of medicines is an important aspect of the professional practice of persons whose names are on the Council's register. It is not solely a mechanistic task to be performed in strict compliance with the written prescription of a medical practitioner. It requires thought and the exercise of professional judgement ...
>
> *NMC 2002, p. 3*

You will need, especially in the beginning of your career, to look things up every time you give them.

- Look things up in the *British National Formulary* (*BNF*) or the *Monthly Index of Medical Specialities* (*MIMS*), or get your own drug handbook (you can get your own copy of the *BNF* if you ask a chemist for a just-out-of-date one!) I like Mosby's *Nurse's Drug Handbook* from the US. It's not cheap but it gives a lot of very useful information.
- Don't ever put something into a patient if you don't know what it is, what it does and what harm it could do. Your patients trust you to keep them safe.
- Always know the side-effects and contraindications (reasons not to give) of any medication. If you aren't sure, don't give it.
- You can help yourself become more familiar by keeping a little notebook and writing down medications, how they are given, what they do and why they are given.

As you gain experience you will become familiar with certain drugs and classes of drugs, and you won't need to look them up every time.

Nurse prescribing

Nurse prescribing is discussed in Appendix 8.

The five rights

There are five basic things you need to remember when giving a medication. If you follow the '5 rights', you shouldn't ever make a medication error:

1. The right patient being given …
2. … the right medication in …
3. … the right dose by …
4. … the right route of administration at …
5. … the right time.

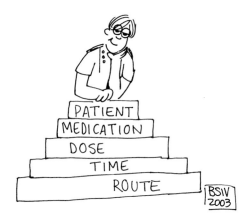

1. The right patient

- Have you correctly identified your patient beyond any doubt?
- Is the patient properly positioned to take this medication?
- Has the patient consented?
- Does the patient understand what they are being given and why?

2. The right medication

- Is it appropriate for this patient to receive this medication? (Are there any contraindications?)
- Does the reason the medication is being given make sense?

- Is the patient allergic?
- Are you sure this is the medication that has been ordered?
- Is it within its 'use by' date?
- Has the prescription been properly written by an authorized person?
- Does the tablet or solution look cloudy, broken down or damaged? If so, double-check – how should it look?
- Are you qualified to give this medication in this way?
- Make sure you don't crush or dissolve capsules or tablets without checking with the pharmacist. Don't mix liquid medications together without checking either.
- Note: some types of controlled medication require two nurses to give them. Because you are not a nurse, you cannot be the 'second' nurse who checks a controlled drug.

3. The right dose

- Have you done, and had double-checked, any calculations and conversions?
- Is the dose within the prescribing guidelines?
- Is it in the right unit?
- How many tablets or units are you giving the patient? If it seems extreme, double-check.

4. The right route of administration

- Are you sure you are putting this in the place it is supposed to be? There have been cases of suppositories being given orally … if you are not *certain*, double-check – don't assume!
- Is this route appropriate for this medication and this patient?
- Do you have patient consent to give this medication in this way?
- Are you qualified to give medication by this route?

5. The right time

- For what time is the medication ordered?

- Is this an appropriate time to give this medication? Will it keep the patient up all night, upset his or her stomach, or interact with other medications?
- If the administration of the medication has been delayed, check before giving to make certain it is still OK to give. Document that it was given late, with the reason and who told you it was still OK to give.

Here are a few examples of how things can go wrong:

- The patient has a potent laxative ordered, in preparation for an investigation. The investigation is cancelled. Do you still give the laxative? After all, it's been ordered!
- Medication is ordered but the patient is NBM (nil by mouth). Do you give the pills?
- The patient is allergic to penicillin, but flucloxacillin has been ordered. Do you give it?
- The patient gets digoxin 0.125 milligrams. The heart rate is 50. Do you give it?
- The patient is taking a medication in the morning but it says to give on an empty stomach at least 1 hour before food. Because of the timing of morning drug rounds and breakfast, the patient might miss breakfast every day. You look up the drug in the *BNF* and it says to give it at bedtime. What do you do?

Each of these examples requires the nurse to know more than what is written on the medication chart. You need to look the medications up and understand why they are being used.

Sometimes you might be asked to 'hide' medications in food or tell a patient a medication is one thing when it is another. This is called 'covert' administration. Although this might be considered necessary, there are legal and ethical issues that you must consider. Before giving medication covertly, speak to your mentor. If you are uncomfortable giving a medication this way, you have a right to refuse.

As a student, you need to make sure that a qualified nurse supervises (stands there and watches) you giving medication, and that this nurse co-signs the medication chart (it is *your* obligation to get this co-signed). If you don't give a medication that is ordered, you should write up the reasons in the medication chart or in the patient's notes. You should also contact the prescriber if you discover a reason why you shouldn't give the medication.

If you find out that a drug has been prescribed improperly, don't just give it because you are a student and you think you don't have the right to challenge. The patient trusts you. You need to contact the prescriber. Perhaps there is a reason the drug has been prescribed to be given a certain way. If so, no harm comes by you questioning. If it was a mistake ... well, wouldn't you rather know for sure before you give the medication? If you ever are unsure of the safety in giving a certain medication, don't give it.

Summary

- Nurses must use good judgement when giving medication.
- Follow the 'five rights' rule.
- Nurses should know as much as possible about the medications they are giving.
- Nurses, even students, have an obligation to question possible errors or mistakes in a prescription.
- Every nurse and student should have a copy of the NMC booklet *Guidelines for the Administration of Medicines*. It is reproduced in Appendix 8.1 at the end of this chapter.

REFERENCES

Gatford J, Phillips N 2002 *Nursing calculations*. Churchill Livingstone, Edinburgh

NMC 2002 Guidelines for the administration of medicines. NMC, London

Appendix 8.1: NMC *Guidelines for the Administration of Medicines*

Guidelines for the Administration of Medicines was first published by the former United Kingdom Central Council for Nursing, Midwifery and Health Visiting [UKCC] in October 2000. In April 2002, this revised edition was published by the new Nursing and Midwifery Council [NMC]. The guidelines themselves remain unchanged and the only textual changes are a small number of minor amendments necessitated by the transfer to the new regulatory body. The NMC will keep these guidelines under review and will notify all registered nurses and midwives in advance of any changes that will lead to the publication of a revised edition.

The NMC Guidelines for the Administration of Medicines

As the regulatory body for nursing and midwifery, the primary function of the Nursing and Midwifery Council [NMC] is public protection through professional standards. One of the most important ways of serving the public interest is through providing advice and guidance to registrants on professional issues. The purpose of this booklet is to establish principles for safe practice in the management and administration of medicines by registered nurses and midwives. As many changes have taken place in relation to medicines management and the way health care is developed in the United Kingdom, it has been necessary to review the advice previously given by the regulatory body on the administration of medicines. Guidelines for the administration of medicines therefore replaces the 1992 document Standards for the administration of medicines. It was reprinted by the NMC in April 2002. However, many of the principles contained in that guidance are of equal relevance today. For example:

> 'The administration of medicines is an important aspect of the professional practice of persons whose names are on the Council's register. It is not solely a mechanistic task to be performed in strict compliance with the written prescription of a medical practitioner. It requires thought and the exercise of professional judgement ...'.

Many government and other agencies are involved in medicines management, from manufacture, licensing, prescribing and dispensing, to administration. An extensive range of guidance on these issues is provided by the relevant bodies. Sources of information are listed on pages 13–14. One of the best sources of advice locally is usually your pharmacist.

As with all NMC guidance, this booklet is neither intended to be a rule book nor a manual. Nor is it intended to cover every single situation that you may encounter during your career. Instead, it sets out a series of guidelines or principles that we hope will enable you to think through the issues and to apply your professional expertise and judgement in the best interests of your patients. It will also be necessary to develop and refer to additional local policies or protocols to suit local needs. Within the document, the word 'patient' is used for convenience to refer to a person receiving medication, irrespective of the environment in which they are residing.

Principles in relation to the prescription

As a registered nurse or midwife, you are accountable for your actions and omissions. In administering any medication, or assisting or overseeing any self administration of medication, you must exercise your professional judgement and apply your knowledge and skill in the given situation.

When administering medication against a prescription written manually or electronically by a registered medical practitioner or another authorized prescriber, the prescription should:

- be based, whenever possible, on the patient's informed consent and awareness of the purpose of the treatment
- be clearly written, typed or computer-generated and be indelible (please refer to the NMC's *Guidelines for Records and Record Keeping*)
- clearly identify the patient for whom the medication is intended
- record the weight of the patient on the prescription sheet where the dosage of medication is related to weight
- clearly specify the substance to be administered, using its generic or brand name where appropriate and its stated form, together with the strength, dosage, timing, frequency of administration, start and finish dates and route of administration
- be signed and dated by the authorized prescriber
- not be for a substance to which the patient is known to be allergic or otherwise unable to tolerate
- in the case of controlled drugs, specify the dosage and the number of dosage units or total course; if in an out-patient or community setting, the prescription should be in the prescriber's own handwriting; some prescribers are subject to handwriting exemption but the prescription must still be signed and dated by the prescriber.

Instruction by telephone to a practitioner to administer a previously unprescribed substance is not acceptable. In exceptional circumstances, where the medication has been previously prescribed and the prescriber is unable to issue a new prescription, but where changes to the dose are considered necessary, the use of information technology (such as fax or e-mail) is the preferred method. This should be followed up by a new prescription confirming the changes within a given time period. The NMC suggests a maximum of 24 hours. In any event, the changes must have been authorized before the new dosage is administered.

Prescribing

Detailed guidance on prescribing is contained in the *British National Formulary* [BNF] and in *Medicines, Ethics and Practice: A Guide for Pharmacists*. Until 1992, prescribing was essentially restricted to doctors and dentists.

Prescribing by nurses and midwives

The *Medicinal Products: Prescription by Nurses Act 1992* and subsequent amendments to the pharmaceutical services regulations allow health visitors and district nurses, who have recorded their qualification on the NMC register, to become nurse prescribers. The preparation for this new area of practice is also included in the appropriate programmes to enable newly-qualified health visitors and district nurses to prescribe.

Practitioners whose prescribing status is denoted on the register and who are approved within their employment setting may prescribe from the *Nurse Prescribers' Formulary*. Nurse and midwife prescribers must comply with the current legislation for prescribing and be accountable for their practice.

Patient group directions (group protocols)

Changes to medicines legislation, which came into effect in August 2000, clarify the law in relation to the supply or administration of medicines under patient group directions, previously termed group protocols. You must follow the guidance supplied by your government health department regarding implementation.

A patient group direction is a specific written instruction for the supply and administration of a named medicine or vaccine in an identified clinical situation. It applies to groups of patients who may not be individually identified before presenting for treatment. Patient group directions are drawn up locally by senior doctors or, if appropriate, by dentists, pharmacists and other health professionals.

They must be signed by a doctor or dentist and a senior pharmacist, both of whom should have been involved in developing the direction, and must be approved by the appropriate health care body.

Dispensing

If, under exceptional circumstances, you are required to dispense, there is no legal barrier to this practice. However, this must be in the course of the business of a hospital and in accordance with a doctor's written instructions. In a dispensing doctor's practice, nurses may supply to patients under a particular doctor's care, when acting under the directions of a doctor from that practice. Dispensing includes such activities as checking the validity of the prescription, the appropriateness of the medicine for an individual patient, assembly of the product, labelling in accordance with legal requirements and providing information leaflets for the patient.

If you, as a registered nurse or midwife, are engaged in dispensing, this represents an extension to your professional practice. The patient has the legal right to expect that the dispensing will be carried out with the same reasonable skill and care that would be expected from a pharmacist.

Principles for the administration of medicines

In exercising your professional accountability in the best interests of your patients, you must:

- know the therapeutic uses of the medicine to be administered, its normal dosage, side effects, precautions and contra-indications
- be certain of the identity of the patient to whom the medicine is to be administered
- be aware of the patient's care plan
- check that the prescription, or the label on medicine dispensed by a pharmacist, is clearly written and unambiguous
- have considered the dosage, method of administration, route and timing of the administration in the context of the condition of the patient and co-existing therapies
- check the expiry date of the medicine to be administered
- check that the patient is not allergic to the medicine before administering it
- contact the prescriber or another authorized prescriber without delay where contra-indications to the prescribed medicine are discovered, where the patient develops a reaction to the medicine, or where assessment of the patient indicates that the medicine is no longer suitable
- make a clear, accurate and immediate record of all medicine administered, intentionally withheld or refused by the patient, ensuring that any written entries and the signature are clear and legible; it is also your responsibility to ensure that a record is made when delegating the task of administering medicine
- where supervising a student nurse or midwife in the administration of medicines, clearly countersign the signature of the student. Some drug administrations can require complex calculations to ensure that the correct volume or quantity of medication is administered. In these situations, it may be necessary for a second practitioner to check the calculation in order to minimize the risk of error. The use of calculators to determine the volume or quantity of medication should not act as a substitute for arithmetical knowledge and skill.

It is unacceptable to prepare substances for injection in advance of their immediate use or to administer medication drawn into a syringe or container by another practitioner when not in their presence. An exception to this is an already established infusion which has been instigated by another practitioner following the principles set out above, or medication prepared under the direction of a pharmacist from a central intravenous additive service and clearly labelled for that patient.

In an emergency, where you may be required to prepare substances for injection by a doctor, you should ensure that the person administering the drug has undertaken the appropriate checks as indicated above.

Midwives should refer to the NMC's *Midwives Rules and Code of Practice* for specific additional information.

Aids to support concordance (compliance aids)

Self-administration from dispensed containers may not always be possible for some patients. If an aid to concordance is considered necessary, careful attention should be given to the assessment of the patient's suitability and understanding of how to use an appropriate aid safely. However, all patients will need to be regularly assessed for continued appropriateness of the aid. Ideally, any concordance aid, such as a monitored dose container or a daily/weekly dosing aid, should be dispensed, labelled and sealed by a pharmacist.

Where it is not possible to get a concordance aid filled by a pharmacist, you should ensure that you are able to account for its use. The patient has a right to expect that the same standard of skill and care will be applied by you in dispensing into a concordance aid as would be applied if the patient were receiving the medication from a pharmacist. This includes the same standard of labelling and record keeping. Compliance aids, which are able to be purchased by patients for their own use, are aids that are filled from containers of dispensed medicines. If you choose to repackage dispensed medicines into compliance aids, you should be aware that their use carries a risk of error.

Self-administration of medicines

The NMC welcomes and supports the self-administration of medicines and the administration of medication by carers wherever it is appropriate. However, the essential safety, security and storage arrangements must be available and, where necessary, agreed procedures must be in place. For the hospital patient approaching discharge, but who will continue on a prescribed medicines regime on the return home, there are obvious benefits in adjusting to the responsibility of self-administration while still having access to professional support. It is essential, however, that where self-administration is introduced, arrangements are in place for the safe and secure storage of the medication, access to which is limited to the specific patient. Where self-administration of medicines is taking place, you should ensure that records are maintained appropriate to the environment in which the patient is being cared for.

It is also important that, if you are delegating this responsibility, you ensure that the patient or carer/care assistant is competent to carry out the task. This will require education, training and assessment of the patient or carer/care assistant and further support if necessary. The competence of the person to whom the task has been delegated should be reviewed periodically.

Complementary and alternative therapies

Complementary and alternative therapies are increasingly used in the treatment of patients. Registered nurses and midwives who practise the use of such therapies must have successfully undertaken training and be competent in this area (please refer to the *Code of Professional Conduct*). You must have considered the appropriateness of the therapy to both the condition of the patient and any co-existing treatments. It is essential that the patient is aware of the therapy and gives informed consent.

Management of errors or incidents in the administration of medicines

It is important that an open culture exists in order to encourage the immediate reporting of errors or incidents in the administration of medicines. If you make an error, you must report it immediately to your line manager or employer. Registered nurses and midwives who have made an error, and who have been honest and open about it to their senior staff, appear sometimes to have been made the subject of local disciplinary action in a way that might discourage the reporting of incidents and, therefore, be potentially detrimental to patients and the maintenance of standards.

The NMC believes that all errors and incidents require a thorough and careful investigation at a local level, taking full account of the context and circumstances and the position of the practitioner involved. Such incidents require sensitive management and a comprehensive assessment of all the circumstances before a professional and managerial decision is reached on the appropriate way to proceed. If a practising midwife makes or identifies a drug error or incident, she should also inform her supervisor of midwives as soon as possible after the event.

The NMC supports the use of local multi-disciplinary critical incident panels, where improvements to local practice in the administration of medicines can be discussed, identified and disseminated. When considering allegations of misconduct arising from errors in the administration of medicines, the NMC takes great care to distinguish between those cases where the error was the result of reckless or incompetent practice or was concealed, and those that resulted from other causes, such as serious pressure of work, and where there was immediate, honest disclosure in the patient's interest. The NMC recognizes the prerogative of managers to take local disciplinary action where it is considered to be necessary but urges that they also consider each incident in its particular context and similarly discriminate between the two categories described above.

Legislation

There are a number of pieces of legislation that relate to the prescribing, supply, storage and administration of medicines. It is essential that you comply with them. The following is a summary of those that are of particular relevance.

Medicines Act 1968

This was the first comprehensive legislation on medicines in the United Kingdom. The combination of this primary legislation and the various statutory instruments (secondary legislation) on medicines produced since 1968 provides the legal framework for the manufacture, licensing, prescription, supply and administration of medicines.

Among recent statutory instruments of particular relevance to registered nurses and midwives is *The Prescription Only Medicines (Human Use) Order 1997, SI No 1830*. This consolidates all previous secondary legislation on prescription-only medicines and lists all of the medicines in this category. It also sets out who may prescribe them. The sections on exemptions are of particular relevance to midwives, including those in independent practice, and to nurses working in occupational health settings.

The *Medicines Act 1968* classifies medicines into the following categories:

Prescription-only medicines (POMs)

These are medicines that may only be supplied or administered to a patient on the instruction of an appropriate practitioner (a doctor or dentist) and from an approved list for a nurse prescriber. The pharmacist is the expert on all aspects of medicines legislation and should be consulted.

Pharmacy-only medicines

These can be purchased from a registered primary care pharmacy, provided that the sale is supervised by the pharmacist.

General sale list medicines (GSLs)

These need neither a prescription nor the supervision of a pharmacist and can be obtained from retail outlets.

Generally, no medication should be administered without a prescription. However, local policies or patient group directions should be developed to allow the limited administration of medicines in this group to meet the needs of patients.

Misuse of Drugs Act 1971

This prohibits the possession, supply and manufacture of medicinal and other products, except where such possession, supply and manufacture has been made legal by the *Misuse of Drugs Regulations 1985*. The legislation is concerned with controlled drugs and categorizes these into five separate schedules. As a registered nurse or midwife, you should be particularly familiar with the regulations concerning schedule 2 medicines such as morphine, diamorphine and pethidine, and schedule 3 drugs such as barbiturates.

If you are responsible for the storage or administration of controlled drugs, you should be aware of the content of the *Misuse of Drugs Regulations 1985* and the *Misuse of Drugs (Safe Custody) Regulations 1973*. Queries are often raised in relation to prescriptions for schedule 2 medicines (controlled drugs). The legislation states that the prescription should:

- be in ink or such as to be indelible, and be signed and dated by the prescriber, issuing it in their usual handwriting with their signature
- specify the dose to be taken and, in the case of a prescription containing a controlled drug which is a preparation, the form and, where appropriate, the strength of the preparation, and either the total quantity (in both words and figures) of the preparation or the number (in both words and figures) of dosage units, as appropriate, to be supplied; in any other case, the total quantity (in both words and figures) of the controlled drug to be supplied.

If you have any queries in relation to the misuse of drugs, or if you are aware of illicit substances being in the possession of a patient, you must refer to and act on local policy and/or appropriate government health department guidance.

Unlicensed medicines

An unlicensed medicine is the term used to refer to a medicine that has no product licence. If an unlicensed medicine is administered to a patient, the manufacturer has no liability for any harm that ensues. The person who prescribes the medicine carries the liability. This may have implications for you in obtaining informed consent.

If a medicine is unlicensed, it should only be administered to a patient against a patient-specific prescription and not against a patient group direction. However, medication which is licensed but used outside its licensed indications may be administered under a patient group direction if such use is exceptional, justified by best practice and the status of the product is clearly described. In addition, you should be satisfied that you have sufficient information to administer the drug safely and, wherever possible, that there is acceptable evidence for the use of that product for the intended indication.

Published by the former United Kingdom Central Council for Nursing, Midwifery and Health Visiting in October 2000
Reprinted by the Nursing and Midwifery Council in April 2002

Sources of information and advice

This is not intended to be a definitive list but simply a guide to some of the organizations which can provide you with additional information and advice in relation to the administration of medicines.

Royal Pharmaceutical Society of Great Britain
1 Lambeth High Street, London SE1 7JN
Telephone 020 7735 9141

The Pharmaceutical Society of Northern Ireland
73 University Street, Belfast BT7 1HL
Telephone 028 90 326 927

Scottish Pharmaceutical General Council
42 Queen Street, Edinburgh EH2 3NH
Telephone 0131 467 7766

Office of the Chief Pharmacist
Department of Health, Richmond House, 79 Whitehall, London SW1A 2NS
Telephone 020 7210 5761

Home Office
50 Queen Anne's Gate, London SW1H 9AP
Telephone 020 7273 3474

Medicines Control Agency
Market Towers, 1 Nine Elms Lane, London SW8 5NQ
Telephone 020 7273 0000

Medical Devices Agency
Hannibal House, Elephant and Castle, London SE1 6TQ
Telephone 020 7972 8124

NMC Professional Advice Service
23 Portland Place, London W1B 1PZ
Telephone 020 7333 6541/6550/6553 fax 020 7333 6538
e-mail advice@nmc-uk.org
www.nmc-uk.org

Useful publications

The *British National Formulary* and the *Nurse Prescribers' Formulary* are published jointly by the British Medical Association and the Royal Pharmaceutical Society of Great Britain. Copies are available from the Pharmaceutical Press, PO Box 151, Wallingford, Oxfordshire OX10 8QU.

The *Monthly Index of Medical Specialities* [MIMS] is available from MIMS Subscriptions, PO Box 43, Ruislip, Middlesex HA4 0YT, telephone 020 8845 8545 or fax 020 8845 7696.

The *Review of Prescribing, Supply and Administration of Medicines: A Report on the Supply and Administration of Medicines under Group Protocols*, (Crown I) (Department of Health, London, April 1998) was published under cover of Health Service Circular (HSC) 1998/051 in England; Management Executive letter (MEL) (98)29 in Scotland; Welsh Health Circular (WHC) (98)27 in Wales, and by each Chief Professional Officer to their respective professional groups in Northern Ireland. Copies are available from the NHS response line on 0541 555 455. The *Review of Prescribing, Supply and Administration of Medicines: Final Report* (Crown II)

(Department of Health, London 1999) is available from the same source. *Medicines, Ethics and Practice: A Guide for Pharmacists* is published annually and is available from the Royal Pharmaceutical Society of Great Britain (see above for contact details). Copies of all legislation cited in this publication are available from local branches of The Stationery Office. The drugs manufacturer's data sheet is also an essential source of information. For a list of current NMC publications, please refer to our website at www.nmc-uk.org or write to the Publications Department at the NMC's address or by e-mail at publications@nmc-uk.org.

Reproduced with permission of the NMC.

Appendix 8.2: UKCC *Statement on the Covert Administration of Medicines*

UKCC position statement on the covert administration of medicines – disguising medicine in food and drink

Introduction

1. This statement has been prepared to explain the UKCC's position on the covert administration of medicines, or disguising medication in food or drink. It supplements, and should be read in conjunction with, the UKCC's *Guidelines for the Administration of Medicines*, published in October 2000.
2. The UKCC recognizes that this is a complex issue that has provoked widespread concern. It involves the fundamental principles of patient and client autonomy and consent to treatment, which are set out in common law and statute and underpinned by the Human Rights Act 1998.

Overview

3. This position statement seeks to deliver guidance on the covert administration of medicine and the deceptive nature of this practice. This should not be confused with the administration of medicines against someone's will, which in itself may not be deceptive, but may be unlawful.
4. Disguising medication in the absence of informed consent may be regarded as deception. However, a clear distinction should always be made between those patients or clients who have the capacity to refuse medication and whose refusal should be respected, and those who lack this capacity. Among those who lack this capacity, a further distinction should be made between those for whom no disguising is necessary because they are unaware that they are receiving medication, and others who would be aware if they were not deceived into thinking otherwise.

5. The UKCC's *Code of Professional Conduct* requires each registered nurse, midwife and health visitor to act at all times in such a manner as to justify public trust and confidence. Registered practitioners are personally account-able for their practice and, in the exercise of professional accountability, must work in an open and co-operative manner with patients/clients and their families, foster their independence and recognize and respect their involvement in the planning and delivery of care.

6. As a general principle, by disguising medication in food or drink, the patient or client is being led to believe that they are not receiving med-ication, when in fact they are. The registered nurse, midwife or health visitor will need to be sure that what they are doing is in the best inter-ests of the patient or client, and be accountable for this decision.

7. The registered practitioner will need to ascertain whether they have the support, or otherwise, of the rest of the multi-professional team, and make their own views clear. It is inadvisable for the nurse, midwife or health vis-itor to make a decision to dispense medication in this way in isolation.

8. Even with completed risk assessments and guidelines, and following the involvement of all relevant parties, it is imperative that good record keep-ing should support duty of care arguments.

General principles

9. The best interests of the patient or client are paramount. The interests of the practitioner, team, or organization should not determine any decision to administer medicines. In drafting a local policy or protocol on covert medication, health professionals should seek advice from their trust's or service provider's legal advisors. There should be a framework within every clinical setting for open multi-professional discussion and access to legal advice if necessary. These discussions and any possible resulting action must be documented in the current care plan.

10. The UKCC believes that local policies or procedures should be revised and developed in accordance with this position statement and the *Code of Professional Conduct*.

The general framework of professional conduct

11. The guidance given in this position statement is presented on the under-standing that registered practitioners administering medicines do so within the boundaries of the UKCC's:
    - Code of professional conduct, 1992
    - The scope of professional practice, 1992
    - Guidelines for professional practice, 1996
    - Guidelines for the administration of medicines, 2000
    - Guidelines for records and record keeping.

12. Every registered practitioner involved in this practice should reflect on the treatment aims of disguising medication. Such treatment must be necessary in order to save life or to prevent a deterioration or ensure an improvement in the patient's or client's physical or mental health. In other words, it must be in the best interests of the patient or client.

13. Registrants involved in the practice of administering medicines covertly should be fully aware of the aims, intent and implications of such treatment. Disguising medication in order to save life, prevent a deterioration, or ensure an improvement in the person's physical or mental health, cannot be taken in isolation from the recognition of the rights of the person to give consent. It may, in such situations, be necessary to administer medicines covertly, but it is worth bearing in mind that, in some cases, the only proper course of action may be to seek the permission of the court to do so.

14. Some forms of forced or disguised medication are recognized by law, for example, if a person is lawfully detained under a section of the relevant mental health legislation.

Consent

15. Every adult must be presumed to have the mental capacity to consent or refuse treatment, including medication, unless he or she:

- is unable to take in and retain the information about it provided by the treating staff, particularly as to the likely consequences of refusal
- or is unable to understand that information
- or is unable to weigh up the information as part of the process of arriving at a decision. The assessment of capacity is primarily a matter for the treating clinicians, but practitioners retain a responsibility to participate in discussions about this assessment.

16. Where adult patients or clients are capable of giving or withholding consent to treatment, no medication should be given without their agreement. For that agreement to be effective, the patient or client must have been given adequate information about the nature, purpose, associated risks and alternatives to the proposed medication. A competent adult has the legal right to refuse treatment, even if a refusal will adversely affect his or her health or shorten his or her life. Therefore, registered nurses, midwives and health visitors must respect a competent adult's refusal as much as they would his or her consent. Failure to do so may amount not only to criminal battery or civil trespass, but also to a breach of their human rights. The exception to this principle concerns treatment authorized under the relevant mental health legislation.

17. When a patient or client is considered incapable of providing consent, or where the wishes of the mentally incapacitated patient or client appear to

be contrary to the best interests of that person, the registered practitioner should provide an objective assessment of the person's needs and proposed care or treatment. He or she should consult relevant people close to the patient or client, such as relatives, carers and other members of the multi-disciplinary team, and respect any previous instructions that the patient or client gave.

18. In some cases the patient or client may have indicated consent or refusal at an earlier stage, while still competent, in the form of a living will or advance statement. Where the patient's or client's wishes are known, practitioners should respect them, provided that the decision in the living will or advance statement is clearly applicable to the present circumstances and there is no reason to believe that the patient or client has changed their mind. The ultimate decision to administer medicines covertly must be one that has been informed and agreed by the team caring for the patient or client.

19. Nobody, not even a spouse, can consent for someone else, although the views of family and close friends may be helpful in clarifying a patient's or client's wishes and establishing his or her best interests.

20. The administration of medicines to patients or clients who lack the capacity to consent and who are unable to appreciate that they are taking medication (unconscious patients or clients, for example) should not need to be carried out covertly. If such patients recover awareness, their consent should be sought at the earliest opportunity.

21. A patient or client may be mentally incapacitated for various reasons. These may be temporary reasons, such as the effect of sedatory medicines, or longer term reasons such as mental illness, coma or unconsciousness. It is important to remember that capacity may fluctuate, sometimes over short periods of time, and should therefore be regularly reassessed by the clinical team treating the patient or client.

Patients or clients with mental illness

22. For patients or clients detained under the relevant mental health legislation, the principles of consent continue to apply to any medication for conditions not related to the mental disorder for which they have been detained. The assessment of their capacity to consent to or refuse such medication therefore remains important. This assessment of capacity to make a decision applies equally to those people with a learning disability who may not have a mental illness. However, in relation to medication for the mental disorder for which the patient or client has been detained, medication can be given against a patient's wishes during the first three

months of a treatment order or afterwards if sanctioned by a Second Opinion Approved Doctor (SOAD).

23. The principle of second opinion should be maintained for informal patients as this would be a sound endorsement of good practice and make it easier to defend. This second opinion is provided within the legislation by medical practitioners appointed by the appropriate statutory mental health commission to provide second opinions on treatment under part VI of the Act. They are known as Second Opinion Appointed Doctors (SOAD).

24. As previously stated, mental illness might cause temporary or fluctuating incapacity. This reinforces the need for regular re-assessment.

Children

25. It cannot be assumed that children are unable to give consent. It is important that both legal and professional principles governing consent are applied equally to all, whatever the health care setting, but with the following significant restrictions:

    - Children under the age of 16 are generally considered to lack the capacity to consent to or refuse treatment, including medication. The right to do so remains with the parents, or those with parental responsibility, unless the child is considered to have significant understanding and intelligence (sometimes referred to as the Fraser guidelines, formerly Gillick competence) to make up his or her own mind about it. Children of 16 or 17 are presumed to be able to consent for themselves, but the refusal of a child of any age may be overridden by the parents or those with parental responsibility. In exceptional circumstances, this may involve seeking an order from the court or making the child a ward of court.

    - The Legal Capacity (Scotland) Act 1991 sets out the current position on the legal capacity of children, including giving or withholding consent to treatment. The law is broadly similar to that in England and Wales. However, one important difference is that a parent's consent cannot override a refusal of consent by a competent child. In Scotland a child under the age of 16 has the legal capacity to consent to his or her own treatment where, according to the act, ' ... in the opinion of the qualified medical practitioner attending him/her, he/she is capable of understanding the nature and possible consequences of the procedure or treatment.'

The covert administration of medicines

26. The covert administration of medicines is only likely to be necessary or appropriate in the case of patients or clients who actively refuse medication

but who are judged not to have the capacity to understand the consequences of their refusal.

27. The UKCC recognizes that there may be certain exceptional circumstances in which covert administration may be considered to prevent a patient or client from missing out on essential treatment. In such circumstances and in the absence of informed consent, the following considerations may apply:

- The best interests of the patient or client must be considered at all times.
- The medication must be considered essential for the patient's or client's health and well being, or for the safety of others.
- The decision to administer a medication covertly should not be considered routine, and should be a contingency measure. Any decision to do so must be reached after assessing the care needs of the patient or client individually. It should be patient- or client-specific, in order to avoid the ritualized administration of medication in this way.
- There should be broad and open discussion among the multi-professional clinical team and the supporters of the patient or client, and agreement that this approach is required in the circumstances. Those involved should include carers, relatives, advocates, and the multi-disciplinary team (especially the pharmacist). Family involvement in the care process should be positively encouraged.
- The method of administration of the medicines should be agreed with the pharmacist.
- The decision and the action taken, including the names of all parties concerned, should be documented in the care plan and reviewed at appropriate intervals.
- Regular attempts should be made to encourage the patient or client to take their medication. This might best be achieved by giving regular information, explanation and encouragement, preferably by the team member who has the best rapport with the individual.
- There should be a written local policy, taking into account these professional practice guidelines.

Clinical supervision

28. Clinical supervision enables the registered nurse, midwife or health visitor to develop a deeper understanding of what it is to be an accountable practitioner and to link this to the reality of practice. The UKCC recommends that a practice dilemma such as the covert administration of medicines be discussed in this context.

Further information

29. Enquiries should be directed to Joe Nichols, Professional officer, mental health and learning disabilities nursing, on direct telephone 020 7333 6546. Contact the NMC or the NMC website for further information.

September 2001

Reproduced with permission of the NMC.

9

Reading and Understanding Research

❢ I was intimidated by nursing research: it was full of complicated sounding things like 'statistics' and 'sampling'. Now that I understand the process a bit better, I can use research in my assignments and in my practice. ❞

Second-year student nurse

WHY IS RESEARCH IMPORTANT TO EVIDENCE-BASED PRACTICE?

'OK,' I hear you asking, 'why do I need to know this?' You need to be aware of current research firstly because the NMC requires nurses to perform what is called evidence-based practice – that is, nurses must base what they do on current research that shows that the approach/treatment actually works. Also, most nursing courses have a requirement that you are at least able to critique, if not write, a piece of research. And, thirdly, because when you go for jobs beyond the basic entry-level staff nurse, you will need to show that you are aware of current research and use it to inform your practice.

You will probably use research in two basic ways:

1. to inform your practice and the practice in your clinical environment
2. to prepare for exams and assignments (or interviews).

There are two different types of research, and these tell you different kinds of things:

1. **Quantitative research** is more reliable for things that need to be measurable. If the research is about the best wound-care product it would tell you which wounds healed the fastest and had the lowest level of infection.

2. **Qualitative research** gives insight into thoughts, feelings and experiences. For example, when considering the question 'How do patients feel about larval therapy (maggots)?' it is less important to know that *x*% said they would never try it than to know *why* they didn't want to try it. Then, as a nurse, you could use the research to help you find a way to help *your* patients.

In evidence-based practice, you should constantly be asking yourself: 'Is this the best way?' Research can help you answer that question. But it's not as simple as finding one paper that says, 'Yes, it is the right way'. You have to decide if you are going to believe what the research has to say.

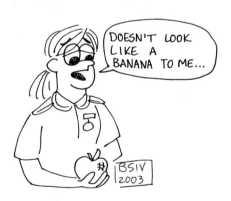

Don't *ever* take for granted *anything* you read. Just because it's published in a book doesn't mean it's absolutely true! It's up to you to decide what you can believe in and what you can't.

Evidence-based practice doesn't mean accepting whatever falls out of the first book you get your hands on – it means knowing that the evidence you are using is credible and reliable. Even you, a nursing student, have to be prepared to critically analyse your evidence base.

RESEARCH BASICS

Let's compare the two basic types of research:

	Qualitative	Quantitative
Sample size	Usually small (10–20). Each person gives a lot of data	Usually large (100+) Each person gives a smaller, more specific amount of data
Reported using:	Narration and excerpts; the data is usually narrative	Statistics, tables, charts; the data is measurable
Gathered through:	Talking, interviewing, group discussions and open-ended questions	Questionnaires with set answers, reviews of data and demographical information, measurements
Replicable?	Not specifically	Yes

Now let's look at an example:

Question	Qualitative research	Quantitative research
What kinds of people become nurses?	Caring people, thoughtful people, people with strong backs, people who like dealing with other people, women	50% of nursing students are over the age of 30; 70% are women. Of 2000 people questioned, 42% said nurses were caring people*

* These results are made up just to give an example.

See the difference? Knowing the type of research lets you know what kind of data the research was based on, and what kinds of evidence the research will give you.

Now try to identify the research type from the research question:

1. This research plans to explore the experiences of pre-registration students during their first clinical placement.
2. This research will determine the average class size of pre-registration nursing students in England.
3. This research will discuss the available sizes of hydrocolloid dressings available to independent nurse prescribers.

Number 1 is qualitative research – it is looking at feelings and experiences; 2 is quantitative research – it is looking at data that can be measured; and 3 is also quantitative research, even though it says it will 'discuss', because it is looking at data that can be measured. To understand research, you also need to know how to dissect a research paper.

READING RESEARCH CRITICALLY

Although research articles can be laid out in many different formats, they almost always contain the same sections. As you read through these sections you will need to ask yourself certain questions. Remember: your goal is to determine if this research is appropriate for you to use as evidence to base your decisions and your practice on. You need to think critically!

Author

When you are looking for research the first thing you will see is the name of the author, the title of the article and the journal where it is published. These things start to tell you about the nature of the research. First, you need to establish that the author is a credible person, who has the background and education to write research / a paper of this type. Ask yourself:

- Does the author have academic and/or research credentials?
- If you do a search for that author, what other kinds of papers and research come up?
- Where does the author work? What is his or her expertise?

Title

This should sum up what the research is about. The title should give a clear indication of the nature of the paper.

- What expectations does the title give you about the nature and content of the article?
- Is it clear and specific?
- Does it make sense?

Go back to the title after you have read the paper and compare what you *thought* it meant before you read the paper. Is there a difference?

Where is the article? The name of the journal

Some journals have a reputation for being very academic and reliable. Others may be seen as less academic and more 'fluffy'. You need to think about the kind of journal you found the research in.

- Is this a credible journal (e.g. was there an article in it about how to cut the toenails of the Beast of Bodmin?).
- What is the journal's audience?
- Is it the journal of a particular group or organization, and could that present a bias?

If an article on the healing properties of honey appears in a journal published by the Society of Beekeepers, you might worry that it could be biased because the people publishing the journal have something to gain by having you think that honey is good. The same article published in the *Journal of Advanced Wound Care* would have more credibility because the people publishing it have nothing to gain by your buying honey. In the same light, an article about building beehives published in the *Wound Care Journal* wouldn't be taken seriously by beekeepers (assuming they ever see it!).

Abstract and key words

The abstract and key words help you get a general idea of what the article is about. The key words are listed to help you find the article when you do an electronic search. If you want to find similar articles, search using the key words.

Read the abstract before you read the paper. Then, after you read the paper, compare what the research said with what the abstract promised it would say. Did they match? Did the abstract leave anything important out?

Introduction

The introduction introduces the research question and sets the scene for what will come. You should ask yourself:

- Why did someone feel this was important to research?
- How and why is this relevant to nursing practice?
- Is the need for this research supported?
- Is the research question sensible?
- Is the research question something that is answerable?
- Is this the right kind of research for this kind of question?

Literature review

The introduction often contains a literature review. Doing a literature review is a real art. In it you will find other information and research available about the topic under investigation. To learn to do a literature review you will need to read a book about research (there are some suggestions in the Useful Books, Journals and Other Resources chapter at the end of this book). To review the literature, you need to ask yourself:

- Is this new research a replication of old research?
- What has changed since any old research was done on this issue?
- Are the sources cited in the literature review accessible and credible?
- If there are other sources (which you would know about because you did a search), why haven't they been used?
- Is the literature review biased in any way?

You will need to look at the different sources listed in the literature review in the same way you are looking at the piece of literature in which they are contained – that is, critically. If the literature review is based on shoddy and unreliable sources, it could affect the credibility of the research overall.

Method

This area talks about how the research is done. It should be broken down into more specific subsections. If it isn't, you might want to question why. The next few headings can all come under the heading 'Method':

Sample

This explains who participated in the research, how they were found and why they were chosen. You need to look critically at the sample size and selection.

- Who was chosen to participate? Why?
- Were these appropriate sources?

- Is the method of choosing the sample appropriate?
- How long ago was this done? Has anything significant changed since then?
- Is confidentiality maintained?
- Is the sample size too big, or too small?
- Does the size and type of sample match the type of research being done?

Also, think: if you were a member of the sample, would you feel that the research adequately represented what you said and did?

Ethical issues

What ethical considerations are there, and how are they addressed? Remember your ethical principles. Research must be presented accurately but participants have a right to confidentiality.

To protect research participants and to ensure quality research, researchers must bring their proposals to an 'ethics committee'. This committee will look at the research question, the planned sample and methodology, and look at the ways that the research plans on resolving any ethical issues raised during or by the research. This includes protecting the confidentiality of the participants.

- Did the author get ethical approval for this work?
- Did participants give consent?
- How did the author find participants?
- Were there any special considerations for the participants?
- How is participant confidentiality protected?
- Did the author have permission, from organizations, workplaces, etc. to do this research?

Are there any issues raised as a result of this research that have ethical considerations? For example, if the research was into the use of a particular medication and it was found early on that a particular dose of this medication was dangerous, did they continue the research using that dose or stop it?

Data collection

How was the data collected – what method of collection was used and how did it work? Data can be collected in many different ways, which are usually called 'tools'. Some tools could be interviews, questionnaires or focus groups. This section should explain the tool that the researcher used. You could then look that tool up in a research text to find out if the researcher used and applied it properly.

- Is this an appropriate way to collect this data?
- Is the tool reliable?
- Is the tool used properly?
- Does the research type support the tool? For example, if this is quantitative research and a survey was used, did it really produce the right kind of data for that method?

Using an inappropriate tool can skew the data, so it is important that you are critical about the way the data was collected.

Validity/reliability/rigour

'Validity' and 'reliability' are terms used to discuss how credible the data is. Data collected for quantitative research is held to a very specific standard: researchers must prove that the numbers and statistics being presenting could be replicated in another study. This proves that the information they are presenting is accurate and correct. Qualitative research doesn't have to prove it can be replicated, in fact, it is expected that qualitative research could not be specifically repeated. Qualitative researchers prove their data is accurate and correct by showing they were rigorously using the correct methods and took every possible opportunity to remove any researcher bias.

To determine if the research is reliable, you need to ask:

- Does the data all make sense?
- If the data is based on any other sources, are they credible sources?
- How has the reliability of the data been tested?

- Could this study be replicated with comparable results?
- Are there any assumptions being made?

Results/discussion

This is where the researcher tells you the results of the study. The researcher will refer back to statistics and information from the sections that have come before. To make an analysis of this section, you need to ask:

- Does it make sense?
- Is it useful?
- Does it match with the title and the abstract?
- How do these findings compare with the literature review? Is there anything significant in literature *not* included in the review?
- Are the statistics reported accurately? Do they match?
- Are findings reported in a way that appears biased?
- Do the tables, graphs and statistics actually tell you anything?
- Do the data collection methods and the data that is presented match?

Compare what you find in the summary with what the title, abstract and introduction said. Does it all go together or does it seem like they are talking about different things?

Summary

The summary wraps up the research. It gives conclusions, which may include recommendations or suggestions. It may suggest areas for further study. It might highlight any particular problems or obstacles the researcher encountered. It should answer the research question. Ask yourself:

- Does it make sense?
- Has the question been answered?

- Does it offer ideas for the way forward or to change/reinforce practice?
- Are there areas of future work that should be done as a result of this research?

After the summary come the parts that compare to the movie credits – you know, the parts that scroll by too fast and that no one really looks at anyway because they are trying to dig the popcorn out of their shoes as they leave the cinema. Well, it pays to look at these areas when you are critiquing research.

Acknowledgements

This section tells you if the research was sponsored or done on behalf of anyone else. You can find out if there could have been a bias in the research. Which would you find more credible: research that has been sponsored by the makers of product *x* about how product *x* is the best wound dressing, or the same research offered by the tissue viability department of a teaching hospital? So ask yourself:

- Did the supporter(s) of the research have a vested interest in its outcome?

Referencing

References from the text of the article:

- Were any references left out?
- Does the author often reference him- or herself?
- Are these the sources that you would have used?
- How old are the sources? Are they outdated?
- Are they obscure, difficult-to-find sources?

If you are worried that the article could be biased, get hold of a couple of the sources. Does the way they present their data match the way they have been presented in your research?

APPROACHING RESEARCH

When reading research, read the title, abstract, discussion and summary first. If the material is not relevant or useful to you, drop it. This will save you from wading through paragraphs of methodology and design only to find out that the material doesn't really apply to you.

Some hints for better grades:

- **Do research on your research.** Look-up the author in CINAHL, Ovid, BNI or even just in the library. What else has he or she written? Does this add to or detract away from his or her credibility? Can you use anything else this researcher has written in your critique or support of this piece of work?
- **Do your own literature search.** Look-up related articles from the key words listed. Did the researcher leave out things that look to you as though they should have been included? Is there any newer research than this piece? If you need help learning to do literature searches, look in the library or learning resource centre. There should be information and probably even a friendly person who can help you learn to access the different resources available. Get a good study skills book (like the one by Maslin-Prothero, which is listed in the Useful Books, Journals and Other Resources chapter at the end of this book) to help you.
- **Think about your practice.** Is there something you wish the research had given you but didn't? Is the information it gave you practical?
- **Be a critical reader.** Don't automatically believe everything someone says just because they wrote it down and researched it. Being a good nurse means thinking critically.

If you want to learn to *do* research, some of the books in the Useful Books, Journals and Other Resources chapter at the end of this book can help. But even if you never plan to research anything, it is essential that you can read research critically. Your ability to base your practice in evidence means you need to be able to tell good evidence from bad.

Reflective Practice and Portfolios

10

> ❝ I am so reflective now, I glow in the dark! ❞
> *Post-registration nursing student*

WHAT IS REFLECTION?

Reflection is the process through which you look at yourself and your practice objectively. It is the way you integrate theory and practice, and the way you grow and mature as a professional and as a person. It's how you transform yourself from a student into a nurse, and later how you transform yourself into an expert and competent practitioner. It's also how you prove that evolution to others like tutors, mentors and the NMC.

Reflection is not a process that you do just once – from now on it needs to become an active and ongoing part of your life as a nurse. It can be done on paper and, as such, can be used as proof for assignments. It should also be something you do in your head.

I want you to imagine something …

You are going out to a very important dinner. As you look in the mirror, you notice that your hair is messy and there is a giant stain on the front of your top. Do you:

- *Shave your head, rip off your clothes, wear a hessian sack and a rope around your waist, and hide from the world by moving into a cave on a deserted island off the coast of Sicily so no one will ever know about what a mess you have been.*
- *Go out looking a mess and lie to all your friends that the stain just got there and that your hair is a new trendy style.*
- *Go out looking the way you are without caring how you look.*
- *Fix the hair, change the top, check the mirror again and go out with confidence that you now look your best.*

I hope you would just fix what you saw was wrong and get on with a great night! That's what reflection is all about. Looking at yourself honestly and objectively, seeing what is wrong, fixing it and carrying on. It's an ongoing process.

And you don't just look in the mirror once a day – you check how you look when you have a chance and you look in the mirror when:

- you try on new clothes
- get your hair cut
- you have eaten – to make sure that those little green bits don't stay stuck in your teeth
- you are facing something (or someone!) important that you want to look your best for
- something happens that you know has messed up your appearance, to see how bad it is.

It's the same with reflection. You reflect on your practice and on your skills when:

- you learn something new
- something has changed – a new placement area, new mentor, new module

- you have done something and you want to make certain you did everything the right way and for the right reasons
- you want to prove you are competent, have learned, or have gained skills, knowledge or experience
- you make a mistake, want to learn from it and prevent a similar mistake from happening again.

Reflection is not about:

- blaming anyone, yourself or anyone else
- berating yourself
- being overly critical
- complaining
- being superficial and holding back what you are really thinking and feeling.

Reflection *is* about:

- gaining confidence in what you do well
- recognizing when you could have done better
- learning from your mistakes
- learning about yourself and your behaviour
- trying to see yourself as others see you
- being self-aware
- changing the future by learning from the past.

OK, time for a story …

My first surgical placement in the UK was on a ward that had a day-case unit. I was asked to help a young man who had his arm in a plaster. He was getting ready to go to theatre to have surgery on his ear. I dutifully filled in the preoperative questionnaire. When I was done I asked him if he needed help getting his johnny on for theatre. (Stay with me here, it gets better.) He looked at me with a shocked and somewhat frightened look, as you can imagine. He said 'But the surgery is on my ear'. I nodded, and in my best therapeutic nursing voice I said 'Yes, but you will be unconscious and we may need to do things to you … '. At this point, his face became absolutely blanched. I knew that something was wrong… so I held up the hospital gown and told him 'Sir, I am American, and where I am from, this is what we call a johnny…' and he blurted out, 'But nurse, a johnny's a condom!'

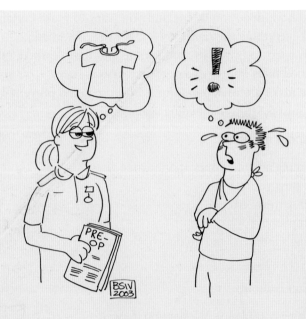

I was speechless for a moment then said, in as dignified a fashion as I could, 'I'll be right back'. I went out to the nurse's station and told sister that the gentleman needed help but would prefer it if one of our male nursing staff assisted him. I then asked if I could go on break. I stood at the end of the corridor and waited to watch his trolley go by on his way to theatre.

I had a storm of feelings going on in my head. Here I was, an experienced nurse, and I had just offered (from the patient's perspective at least) to help him put a condom on. I felt hopeless, like I would never fit in, and that all my nursing experience and skills were useless if I couldn't even communicate. I felt lost.

I felt a hand on my shoulder and one of the staff nurses asked me what was wrong. As best I could, totally humiliated, I told her. And her reaction? She burst out laughing. Here was I, feeling ever so sorry for myself and she was laughing at me! When she stopped laughing she said 'It's time for you to stop being so bloody American-perfect and learn to laugh at yourself!'

It took me back a bit. Here I was trying so hard to be perfect, and she was telling me it was OK to make a huge mistake. It hurt my feelings – but I knew she was right.

I reflected quite a bit on this episode. It wasn't just about making a gaff; it was about re-adjusting my perspectives to this new world in which my nursing would now take place. My first instinct was to run and hide. I was ashamed. I felt that mistakes were beneath me. Through reflection, I identified ways to learn to be a bit more 'British' in the way I said things and it raised my awareness about how my culture (and my coping skills) were perceived by other people. I took a look at the fact that I was quite proud and defensive about my past nursing experience. I can now tell this story for its laughter value and although it still makes me cringe a bit, the experience taught me a lot more than how important it is to call the little dress patients wear to theatre a 'theatre gown'. And that nice Sicilian estate agent gave me back the deposit I put down on the cave I was going to move to. All's well that ends well!

It's going to happen to you; it has happened to every nursing student (and nurse) since time began. You are going to make mistakes. You are going to think those mistakes are irreparable. You're going to convince yourself that your only option is a career in the exciting world of fast food. But, with reflection, you can overcome problems and mistakes and become a self-aware and competent nurse.

REFLECTIVE MODELS

Now that you know how important reflection is to your growth as a professional nurse, you have to learn how to do it. There are numerous models, but the place to start is with Gibbs.

Gibbs' (1988) model of reflection

1. Describe the activity or experience in objective detail.
2. Discuss and explore any feelings you were having at the time of the experience.
3. Evaluate the experience: what really happened? What was good about it? What was bad? What factors contributed to this event?
4. Analyse the experience: what can you learn from it?
5. Conclusion: what could you have done differently? Anything you wish you had done? Wish you hadn't done?
6. Action plan: what can you plan on doing in the future?

John's (1994) model of reflection

1. **Description:** write an objective account of what happened (as in Gibbs). Think 'What are the significant issues I need to pay attention to?' You then go through the experience, using different cues. Each cue should help you to tease the experience apart.

2. **Aesthetics** (the creative, interactive parts of the situation): ask yourself, 'Why did I act as I did? How did my actions affect other people (the patient, my colleagues, other people, myself)? How did other people feel about this situation? How do I know how they feel?'

3. **Personal** (your own thoughts and experiences): 'How was I feeling? What factors influenced me? What was going on in my head?'

4. **Ethics** (the rights and wrongs): 'Did I behave the way I think I should behave? Did I do anything out of character? Anything that makes me feel guilty? Was there anything that made me behave differently than I usually would?'

5. **Empirical** (knowledge and information): 'What information and knowledge did I have or should I have had about this situation?'

6. **Reflexivity** (making sense of things; looking at the past to change the future): 'Does this situation remind me of past situations? What can I do differently in the future? If I did something differently, how would it be different for my patient, my colleagues, others or myself? How do I feel now about this situation? Can I support others better because of this situation and what I have learned? Has this changed the way I behave?'

It doesn't matter which model you use. I have given you the two basic ones here but there are many more basic and advanced ones. You will probably adapt these models to a method that works best for you. It would be a really good idea to read about reflection in more detail. Some books are listed in the Useful Books, Journals and Other Resources chapter at the end of this book, in addition to the sources in the References section at the end of the chapter.

WHY REFLECTION IS IMPORTANT TO PRACTICE

The key to reflection working for you is that you must be *absolutely* honest with yourself. You also have to eliminate the intense desire to involve (blame) other people. 'My mentor ignored me so I went off sick' isn't very useful. 'I was feeling afraid that I wouldn't pass the assessment, and I felt intimidated by my mentor, and I got myself worked up into believing that it would be OK to call in sick because I wanted to avoid having to cope with her' is much better. No one *makes* you do anything: you have to accept responsibility for the choices you make. Focus on *your* thoughts, feelings and reactions. Let other people worry about themselves. You can't change them so don't waste your time trying; just learn from your experiences with them.

You can reflect on anything:

- problems, mistakes and uncomfortable things
- successes and achievements
- journal articles
- classroom sessions
- conversations
- television programmes
- relationships
- placement areas
- how to deal with a particular patient or colleague.

The point is: reflect on experiences that will either help you to grow or will demonstrate that you have grown. Another idea is to look back through your reflections to when you were struggling and to reflect on things that show you have learned from past reflections.

So, it's time to get yourself a notebook and reflect. If you have a particularly good example of how you have changed or what you have learned, put it into your portfolio. It is a good idea to use your notebook as a reflective journal. Develop a pattern for yourself.

- Have a regular time and place to sit and reflect.
- Keep the journal privately, so you can feel free to say whatever you need to without worrying about anyone else.

- When you want to share a reflection, copy it from your journal.
- Look back on past reflections periodically, and then reflect on how you are growing and maturing as a person and as a nurse.
- Get used to reflecting on things in your head as well as on paper.
- Write a reflection when you need to, as well as at your 'usual' time.

Reflection isn't the easiest thing you will do as a student because it requires you to face some things that we all find a bit uncomfortable. Things like 'I rushed because I wanted to leave early', or 'I was impatient because I had other things on my mind.' It's OK. We all have times when we do things for the wrong reasons. It's part of being human and you are allowed to be human, even as a nurse.

Being a good nurse isn't as much about the mistakes you make (because you will make them, trust me!) as about how you learn from and handle those mistakes.

PORTFOLIOS

> ❛ I didn't feel very confident until I looked back over my portfolio – then I saw how much I had accomplished. I didn't realize how far I had come – I'm getting good at being a nurse! ❜
>
> *Third-year student nurse*

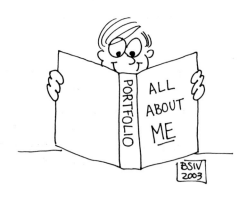

There are two different kinds of portfolio you might be concerned with as a nurse:

1. Student portfolios, both before and after registration. These show evidence of the academic and clinical achievements you need to complete a certain course.
2. Your PREP (post-registration education and practice) portfolio, which shows that you have met the criteria for ongoing registration.

Student portfolios

As a pre-registration student, your student portfolio is there for two main reasons:

1. for you and the uni to keep track of your achievements
2. to see what you still need to get finished.

A side-effect of your student portfolio is that it tells you what is important to you as a nurse. Notice how there is probably an area that talks about your ability to follow aseptic (sterile) technique but nothing about how you make tea.

Pre-registration, it will seem like everyone in the world needs to look at your portfolio. Mentors, personal tutors, even your friends. After you qualify, your portfolio is your own and you don't need to share it with anyone but the NMC. No-one but the NMC can force you to share the content of your portfolio with anyone else.

Your university will supply your student portfolio. It will contain lists of skills (or competencies) that you could develop and practice while on placement. It is up to *you* to know your portfolio, what is included in it and what needs to be done during a specific placement. It is *not* up to your mentor or personal tutor to walk you through the portfolio reminding you of your obligations. It's *your* portfolio: you are in charge of whether or not it gets done.

Look through your portfolio before you go on a placement and try to identify areas that the placement could fulfil. (Yet another reason to do a pre-placement visit and read up about the area in advance!) Plan how to get your needs met and flag up areas you believe you might not achieve during the placement. Share this plan with your mentor and ask for advice and support.

If you are concerned that you are not getting the opportunities you need, speak to your personal tutor and ask for help making your plan.

Keep a photocopy of essential things in your portfolio just in case something happens to it. If you pass a placement, photocopy the part where the mentor says you have passed. If anything ever happens to your portfolio, you still have proof.

Finally, don't see your portfolio as a burden. It's like a baby album – there are portraits of you as a baby nurse, all the way through your development into taking those first steps as a nurse. And, when you are a nurse, your days of keeping a portfolio have only just begun.

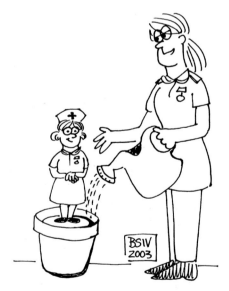

Growing a student nurse

PREP (Post-registration Education and Practice)

Your PREP portfolio is there:

1. for you to keep track of achievements and learning
2. to prove to the NMC that you are a competent practitioner who has kept up with the requirements for registration.

It's a while before you need to produce a PREP portfolio, but you can start to build one when you are a student. You can get a very useful publication called *The PREP Handbook* from the NMC.

You have an obligation to keep yourself up to date in nursing after you qualify and your PREP portfolio is the way you do it. If you start your portfolio as a student it can be very useful when you apply for a nursing job. So, this is what to do:

- Get yourself an A4 binder.
- Type-up your CV as it stood before your nursing course.
- As you get attendance certificates for in-services or trainings, put them into the binder.
- For each assignment you do, write a brief synopsis and record your grade. If you fail, write up another one for the assignment that you submitted that passed and put a reflection about what you did differently!
- Write a brief synopsis about what you have learned in each module you take.
- Write a brief synopsis and reflection about every placement area you have.

Now, when you go to apply for a job, you have a lot of information about how you have prepared yourself to be a nurse. It's not a PREP folder really, because it's pre-registration, but it is the foundation for your eventual PREP. It gets you into the habit of saving things and being on the lookout for proof of your development.

Some of the nurses I know have done their PREP in interesting ways:

- One started going to a gym for her own health, and kept a journal about her feelings so she could work out how to motivate her patients to increase their exercise. She reflected on how learning about exercise and how difficult it is to lose weight gave her more empathy with reluctant patients.

- Another nurse decided to stop smoking and kept a journal, reflecting on what was difficult, how she felt and what was motivating her. She reflected on the process and outlined some ways she could help her patients to stop smoking.
- One elder care nurse did a weekly bank shift in A&E to keep her skills sharp. She reflected on the experiences she had there.
- One nurse reflected on the way nurses behaved on the TV programme *Holby City* and outlined issues with the *Code of Professional Conduct*!

You don't need to work desperately hard to keep up to date. It can be interesting and fun – the key is that you have to keep it relevant. As you go through your daily routines, think about how different things you may see or do could influence the way you do your nursing.

As the time comes for you to complete your course, there will probably be a lecture on how to do your portfolio. The *Nursing Standard* and the *Nursing Times* have both had good articles about portfolio development. Don't wait until the end to start your PREP portfolio: if you start it now, it will be yet another one of those good habits in nursing that you develop.

Summary

- Reflection is a process through which you grow and develop as a person and as a nurse.
- Reflection can be about good and bad things, and shouldn't be about blame or shame.
- Using a reflective model can guide you through the process of reflection more easily.
- You have to be honest with yourself for reflection to be effective.

- Your portfolio is yours, and you are responsible for making sure it is completed.
- You should know the expectations in your portfolio and plan for them to be met through your clinical placements.
- Keep copies of important bits of your student portfolio.
- Start keeping a record of what you do now, to help you start your PREP portfolio and to get into the good habit of paying attention to PREP.

REFERENCES

Gibbs G 1988 Learning by doing: a guide to teaching and learning methods. Oxford Further Education Unit, Oxford

Johns C 1994 Guided reflection. In: Palmer A, Burns S, Bulman C (eds) Reflective practice in nursing. Blackwell Science, Oxford, p 110–130

Legal Issues for Students

11

Nursing is a profession full of legal issues. Having an understanding of those issues as a student will help you develop awareness and good practice for your future career. This is probably going to be a dull chapter – sorry – but these are important issues and I promise that if you wade through this you will find that a lot of it is important and valuable. As always, if you need or want more information, go to the library, ask your personal tutor, check with your mentor, ask at the student union or call your union.

There are many legal issues that you will have to bear in mind as a student and as a nurse but the areas outlined in this chapter are key basics for you. They are things of which you must constantly be aware; they are also things you will be assessed on, so knowing about them will help your grades.

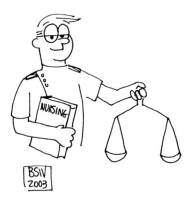

The scales of justice

RECORDS AND RECORD KEEPING

Imagine that you have been brought to court. You are standing in the witness box and an intimidating barrister bellows, 'Student nurse! What did you get for your birthday in 1999?'

Would you be able to remember? You might remember some things but certainly not all, especially the smaller things. Now imagine then that the barrister asks, 'And how were they wrapped? Were there bows? In what order did you open them? What time was it when you opened each item ...'

Would you have the slightest inkling how to answer these questions completely and accurately? Probably not. Even though your birthday comes only once a year and is probably a significant event for you, most people can't remember every detail.

How then would you be able to remember every detail of things you did for patients on an average working day? You have to write them down! Writing things down is the only proof you will have that you did something, recognized something, said something ... if you don't write it down, it never happened.

There are some key points to remember when writing things in patient notes:

- **The notes must be made in a timely manner:** if something significant happens, write it down as soon as possible afterwards.
- **Don't use abbreviations:** except when the abbreviation will be absolutely clear to other readers.

- **Don't use slang or jargon.**
- **Write with a black, non-erasable pen.**
- **Never use Tippex™:** if you must correct an error, put a single line through it, write 'error' above it, initial it, and carry on. If you write an entry in the incorrect patient's notes, cross through it, make another entry below it that says 'The above was entered incorrectly into the incorrect patient's notes' and sign it.
- **Have everything co-signed** by a qualified member of staff.
- **Be clear and specific:** don't write 'Patient in pain. Given meds.' Instead write, 'At 10.00 a.m. patient complained of pain in the surgical area on a scale of 6/10. Given 10 mg of morphine orally at 10.20 a.m. At 11.00 a.m. patient said pain was much better and said no further medication was needed.' Write exactly what you did and when. You might be criticized for writing long notes but, legally, writing clear and specific notes is correct.
- **Be objective and non-judgemental:** write your notes as if the person you are writing about is going to be reading them while sitting next to their solicitor. If you want to convey how someone is acting, simply repeat word for word what they tell you. Don't say someone is 'aggressive or violent'. Instead say, 'Patient states "Get outta my face or I will kill you ..."' If the patient swears, record the swear exactly. This tells others everything they need to know without you being accused of making a judgement. Don't say 'Patient was pouting'. Instead say, 'Patient didn't make eye contact, appeared to be frowning, had arms crossed across chest, didn't answer when spoken to...' Describe what you see and what you hear, and let anyone else reading it make up their own mind!
- **Don't leave blank areas** for other people to fill things in. Put a line through all empty space, then sign your name clearly.
- **Print your name clearly:** if your signature is illegible. While you are a student, note 'student nurse' next to your name.

The following is a summary of the NMC *Guidelines for Records and Record Keeping* (NMC 2002b), which are reproduced in full on pages 192–199.

Summary

- Record keeping is an integral part of nursing and midwifery practice.

- Good record keeping is a mark of the skilled and safe practitioner.

- Records should not include abbreviations, jargon, meaningless phrases, irrelevant speculation and offensive subjective statements.

- Records should be written in terms that the patient or client can easily understand.

- By auditing your records, you can assess the standard of the record and identify areas for improvement and staff development.

- You must ensure that any entry you make in a record can easily be identified.

- Patients and clients have the right of access to records held about them.

- Each practitioner's contribution to records should be seen as of equal importance.

- You have a duty to protect the confidentiality of the patient and client record.

- Patients and clients should own their healthcare records as far as it is appropriate and as long as they are happy to do so.

- The principle of the confidentiality of information held about your patients and clients is just as important in computer-held records as in all other records.

- The use of records in research should be approved by your local research ethics committee.

- You must use your professional judgement to decide what is relevant and what should be recorded.

- Records should be written clearly and in such a manner that the text cannot be erased.

- Records should be factual, consistent and accurate.

- You need to assume that any entries you make in a patient or client record will be scrutinized at some point.

- Good record keeping helps to protect the welfare of patients and clients.

THE DATA PROTECTION ACT

The Data Protection Act (1998) basically boils down to two simple principles:

1. You cannot share any information about someone without his or her permission.
2. Any information you get from someone has to be used in accordance with the reason they gave it to you to begin with.

If, while you are a student, you leave your telephone number with the ward for them to call you if there are any problems, and they use it to call you when your placement has finished to see if you would like to work a shift, this would be seen as a violation of the Data Protection Act unless you told someone it was OK for them to call you for shifts. If they were to give your phone number to another ward, and you didn't know about it and didn't consent, that would also be a violation. Giving your telephone number to a patient's family is certainly a violation!

Basically, people who hold data (called 'data controllers' in the Act) have an obligation to keep the data in accordance with the law and only use it within the correct context.

As a student, you need to be aware that giving out personal information about a patient (or a colleague) could be a problem:

- **Always check with the patient:** 'Mandy, there is a Jane Gardiner on the phone, she says she is your friend and wants to know how you are. What should I tell her?' Perhaps you can't ask the patient; if the person calling is a real friend or family member, he or she will understand if you need to tell them that you can't give them any information. Offer to take a message and pass it on to the patient. If the patient is critically ill, or in serious condition, pass the call to a more senior nurse.

- **Don't ever give out** *any* **staff information:** 'I'm sorry, I cannot give you any information about the off duty or who is working on the ward. You may speak to the ward manager – would you like me to see if she is available?'
- **If you aren't sure what information it is OK to divulge, ask someone.**

You might keep notes from handover, and perhaps even information about patients you have cared for, in your pocket. Don't, it could be used against you. What if someone else, someone who doesn't have the right to that information, finds your scraps of paper? Always destroy, and don't take home, any information about patients.

As we discussed in patient confidentiality, if you need information about a patient for an assignment or your portfolio, you have to make absolutely sure that:

- no-one could identify the patient, or the trust, ward or hospital, from your materials
- you have the patient's consent to use the information.

Not taking care of these two considerations could get you into trouble.

If you feel that, during a placement, your rights under the Data Protection Act have been abused, then you should go to the university, the student union or your union for help.

THE HEALTH AND SAFETY AT WORK ACT

The Health and Safety at Work Act (1974) is a complex one, but there are three basic principles:

1. **Employers:** have an obligation to provide a working environment that does not pose a health or safety risk to employees, and if there are any risks that are present because of the

nature of the work, protective equipment must be supplied by the employer to protect the employee from risk.

2. **Employees:** have an obligation to avoid risk, to be aware of and act in accordance with health and safety protocols and policies, and to notify the appropriate representative of the employer if they become aware of a risk or hazard. If an employee does something that is a violation of the policies, he or she is liable for whatever happens.

3. **Employers and employees:** have an obligation to protect non-employees from risk.

What does this mean for you as a nursing student?

-   You have an obligation to know and follow all relevant health and safety policies, including manual handling, and, as an agent of the employer you have an obligation to be aware of how hazards in the environment could affect other people.
-   If you choose to ignore a policy and either yourself or someone else is harmed, you are in trouble.
-   If you see a hazard and don't tell anyone about it, you could be in trouble, especially if someone else gets hurt.
-   You have a right to have the appropriate protective equipment: aprons, gloves that fit, etc.

Health and safety is a huge issue in the NHS. There are mandatory trainings and policies to follow. Here is how to be certain you are following them:

-   **Stay awake and pay attention** during your mandatory health and safety lectures!
-   **Know how to be safe:** on your first day in a placement area, or on your pre-placement visit if possible, make yourself familiar with fire exits, location of fire extinguishers, how to call for help in an emergency and where any emergency call buttons are. *You must have this information before you do anything else on that ward.*
-   **Find out the location of the health and safety policies.**
-   **Know what you are doing:** if there is any equipment with which you are not familiar, don't use it until you have been properly taught.

- **Protect yourself:** if you need different size gloves, latex-free gloves or need any other personal protection equipment, let someone know and don't work until you have what you need.
- **Be sharp smart:** be aware of the location of sharps boxes and follow sharps disposal policy. Don't *ever* walk around with a sharp in your hand. Don't *ever* recap a syringe. Bring a sharps box with you when you do an injection or use a needle. If you get stuck or stabbed, you *must* report it – your health and career are on the line.
- **Know the environment:** on your pre-placement visit, ask if there are any special health and safety risks in that placement area and, if there are, what procedures are in place for protection. Is there special equipment you will need or need to use? Are there special policies and procedures that will need to be followed? Do any patients require any kind of special care?
- **Be aware of biohazard materials:** handle and dispose of biohazard materials in the appropriate way. If you have any doubts, ask someone to help you. Don't put sharp or potentially sharp (e.g. glass tubes, bottles, IV bags with plastic spikes) items in plastic bin bags. Wash your hands!
- **Wash your hands!!!** I know I've said this already but it is crucial in health and safety.
- **Follow manual handling policy:** if you hurt your back as a student, that's it. Your career is over, you have no recourse to any work injury benefits and you will never be physically the same.
- **Just say no:** if you find yourself put into a situation where you don't feel you can be safe, remove yourself. This includes 'specialing' patients (i.e. supervising one-to-one), lifting, or using equipment you don't know how to use. It also applies when you don't have the protective equipment you need. You have a right to say 'I can't do that'.

It all boils down to protecting yourself, your patients and your colleagues, being aware of risks and of how to protect yourself, and following the policies in place for your protection. Don't ever go beyond the limitations of your role as a student.

DUTY OF CARE

To the average person, someone dressed in a uniform so that he or she looks like a nurse *is* a nurse. That person will expect a certain standard from you and will expect that, as a nurse, you have the knowledge and skills to help. If you are on your way to or from a placement in your uniform you need to be aware that you could be identified as a nurse (most people won't see a difference between a nurse and a student nurse) and expected to help a person in distress. If you let friends, family and neighbours know you are a nursing student then they might also expect you to help if they get into trouble. You need to make it clear that you are a student, not a nurse.

You might be very experienced but you have to accept the limitations of your role as a student. You must make sure that you never act as a nurse without supervision by a qualified nurse. You must make absolutely certain that people know you are a nursing *student* and that being a student is *not* the same as being a nurse.

Duty of care means living up to the standards and expectations held for you, by the NMC and by the general public, as a nurse. It means that you:

- can't just go home when your job is done if there is no one else there
- can't go to lunch or on break if there is no one to cover
- are a nurse 24 hours a day.

Duty of care also means that you have an obligation to uphold the NMC code of professional conduct and to *not* act in a way that could bring discredit to nursing as a profession.

As a student, your duty is less because you are not a nurse but you must remember that patients, their families (and sometimes other professionals) will not necessarily realize that you are a student. It is your responsibility to not take on tasks beyond the scope of your role as a student.

CONSENT

There are two kinds of consent:

1.   implied consent
2.   expressed consent.

Implied consent

Implied consent means you assume, based on circumstances and the situation, that a person would want you to help. If someone is unconscious for example, you don't need to wait until he or she gives you permission to start doing CPR! Implied consent also means that some things are expected of you in your role. Patients expect that you will know how to move and handle them properly; you don't need to get a signed consent form every time you boost them up the bed. If you are in a situation where you know that, although your patient is unable to give expressed consent, they have not already indicated they *don't* want a particular action taken on their behalf, and you believe that a reasonable person would want a certain action taken, then that is implied consent.

Expressed consent

Expressed consent is when a patient actively says 'I want this', knowing the possible complications, side-effects and consequences of the decision. Usually, this means signing a form but in some emergency situations, a doctor or other professional can take consent verbally and ask for those present to witness the consent. Patients should always make *informed consent.*

Informed consent

This means that someone has explained to patients in clear, non-medical language what is happening to them and for what the consent is being sought. It means that patients make decisions about what happens to them with all the information necessary to really understand the impact that decision will have on their life and health.

This means that people who are not able to make competent decisions really can't give consent. Regarding children, the *Guidelines for the Administration of Medicines* (NMC 2002a) states:

> ' Children under the age of 16 are generally considered to lack the capacity to consent to or refuse treatment, including medication. The right to do so remains with the parents, or those with parental responsibility, unless the child is considered to have significant understanding and intelligence [sometimes referred to as the Fraser guidelines, formerly Gillick competence] to make up his or her own mind about it. Children of 16 or 17 are presumed to be able to consent for themselves, but the refusal of a child of any age may be overridden by the parents or those with parental responsibility. In exceptional circumstances, this may involve seeking an order from the court or making the child a ward of court. '

Adults who suffer from an illness or disability that impairs their ability to take in or understand information can have a legal guardian appointed to make decisions for them. You can't assume that family members have a right to make decisions on another person's behalf, even husband and wife. There is no automatic legal right for next of kin to make a decision about a loved one.

Adults with a temporary inability to understand the consequences of a decision or refusal to accept care have to be dealt with carefully. In some cases, their refusal to receive care will be overridden after their inability to make a competent decision is well documented. At other times there will be legal involvement. As a student, you should never allow yourself to get into a situation involving issues of consent because they can get very contentious and, as a student, you really aren't in the position to do anything to help anyway. You should find a qualified nurse who has the accountability and experience to make certain that the patient's rights and health are both protected.

Another issue that involves consent is making sure that a patient really has given informed consent. Before you participate in any procedure for which the patient has given consent, make sure that the patient really does know what is happening. As a student this isn't as much of an issue, but if you have any reason to suspect that the patient doesn't understand what is happening and thus really hasn't given consent, then you have an obligation to bring that concern immediately to a staff nurse, your mentor, a sister or another nurse.

The other side of consent is that patients have the right to say 'No'. Just as you have to make sure you have the patient's consent to do something, you must respect a patient who says 'No'. But, just as consent must be informed consent, any refusal must also be an informed refusal. You have an obligation as a nurse to make absolutely certain that the patient knows the consequences of the decision to refuse care. You also must be able to tell the difference between someone saying 'I don't want that ...' because he or she needs reassurance and someone saying 'You will not do that to me' because he or she really will not allow you to do something. If as a student you are worried that a patient is refusing treatment, step back and don't proceed. Get help and support from your mentor or other nurse. It's something you will deal with more effectively as you gain experience.

ACCOUNTABILITY

Accountability means that you are willing to stand up and say, 'Yes I did that'. Professional accountability means that you are willing for your practice to be examined closely and that you are willing to be honest about what you do and why. It means that you as a nurse can say that you uphold the highest standards of professional nursing care.

As a student, you are not yet 'accountable'. A qualified nurse is accountable under the *Code of Professional Conduct* but you are merely 'responsible' for your behaviour. You must behave in a way

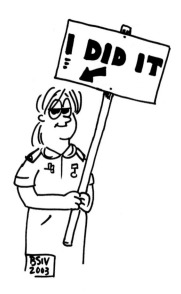

that demonstrates that you are thoughtful and responsible but a qualified nurse must act to a higher standard. You are not yet expected to uphold the highest standards of professional nursing care because you are just a student, and students will make more mistakes than others. That's why you are a student!

An essential aspect of qualified nurses' accountability is that when you as a student work with them, they are accountable for what you may do. That's why they supervise you, because what you do will reflect on them. If you do something under supervision that works out to be the wrong thing (like making a medication error) then the nurse – not you – is the one in trouble as long as you behaved responsibly and within the limits of your education and role as a student. Their training, education and experience gives them a greater level of responsibility.

FITNESS FOR PRACTICE

As a student and as a nurse you have an obligation to be fit for practice. Quite simply, you cannot work as a nurse if you are not emotionally, psychologically or physically fit to do so. Some people are physically injured; others suffer from stress or an illness that interferes with their ability to nurse. Some nurses change to a different type of nursing (for example working for NHS Direct) when illness or injuries make it too difficult for them to work with patients in the clinical area.

You know how you shouldn't drive when you are drunk? Or how you will have to hand back your driving licence if you lose your sight? Well, it's the same in nursing.

If you are ever too stressed, too ill or too injured to work, it is your obligation to let someone know. You must tell your uni and you can make an appointment to see someone in the occupational health department.

You must never attend placement or work a shift when you have been drinking or if you are using recreational drugs. Even some drugs prescribed by your GP could interfere with your judgement. You must be certain that nothing impairs your ability to make the best decisions possible for your patients. Just as you shouldn't drive a car when impaired, so you can't nurse people when you are not able to give your best to care for them. There is no sin in needing to take time to take care of yourself. You can't be the nurse your patients need you to be if you are on the verge of being a patient yourself!

Part of fitness for practice is more than being physically and emotionally well – it's also about being of good character. Can you be a therapeutic nurse who mugs people in her spare time? No. Because, as a nurse, you have access to privileged information and intimate details about people's lives, and because people trust you, you must be a person who is above question. To be fit for practice you must be of sufficiently good character to uphold the trust placed in you.

So, if you get into trouble during your course – are arrested or commit a serious traffic offence – talk to someone at your union or student union and let them know so they can help you make sure it doesn't prevent you from becoming a nurse. Some offences will make it impossible for you to qualify but most things that cause students problems are stupid, silly things that got out of control.

NEGLIGENCE

Negligence is a legal term that means someone didn't do something that should have done, and now that person is liable for the damage the action (or inaction) caused. To be proved negligent, four things must be true:

1. There must be a duty of care present.
2. There must be a breach of that duty (either an act of commission or an act of omission).
3. It must be foreseeable that a breach of duty could cause harm.
4. Harm must result.

We've already talked about duty of care – the expectation that you will behave in a certain way and that you will not abandon a patient – a breach in duty of care means that you either do something wrong, or don't do something you should do. If you breach your duty of care, and you know that a breach could mean that the patient comes to harm, and the patient actually comes to harm, then you are negligent.

One test used when thinking about negligence is the Bolam Test. This basically asks you to think about what most other practitioners just like you would do in a similar situation. If you are acting as most other reasonable practitioners would act in similar circumstances, then you meet the Bolam test and are not negligent.

Negligence is scary, and that's why it's so important for you to understand what your duty of care is. As a student, it's unlikely you would ever be named as negligent because you are working under the direct supervision of a qualified nurse. But if you are ever worried that a potential act or omission could harm someone, you must let your mentor or another nurse know.

BULLYING

Bullying can be a serious issue for students and staff alike. There is no easy way to deal with bullies but there is one thing that you should remember to help you through …

> *It's not your fault if a bully decides to pick on you. There is nothing you could have or should have done differently, it's not your fault and you are not to blame. You are not being bullied because you are weak, and you certainly don't deserve it.*

There are some ways to handle being bullied:

- Recognize that if the bully was really as powerful and important as he or she is trying to make you believe, he or she wouldn't need to resort to bullying to get things done.
- Realize that bullies are really afraid of working with and coping with other people, and act the way they do because they feel inadequate as people.
- Reflect on what happens.
- Don't believe what bullies say. Don't let them into your head.
- Don't try to fix bullies. They are not your problem.

If you feel you are being bullied, go to someone for help immediately. Document what is happening, reflect and try to pinpoint the behaviour that makes you feel bullied. Often, simply standing up to the bully in a gentle way is enough:

'I don't like being spoken to in that way.'

Sometimes, you might even need to say:

'It feels as though you are trying to bully me, and I am not going to tolerate it.'

Sometimes, however, you won't be able to say anything at all. Sometimes the person might be your mentor, or another nurse, colleague, professional or even a patient.

Bullying will destroy your spirit if you allow it to continue. It can erode your confidence and stress you out. It is also wrong and illegal.

So, if you find yourself being bullied, re-read what I said above about it not being your fault. Get help and support from friends, colleagues, at uni, through the student union and through your union. If you see someone else being bullied, support that person and stand up for him or her.

I can't help any more than this in a couple of paragraphs, but what I will tell you is this:

- You don't have to suffer alone; it's important to talk about feeling bullied.
- Bullying is wrong; it is *not* the victim's fault.
- Bullies are people who can't cope with people in the normal, appropriate ways.
- If you are the victim of a bully, there is nothing wrong with you except that you are someone who the bully envies and bullies can't handle someone being good when they feel so bad about themselves.

Remember, document, reflect and go for help as soon as you recognize there is a problem – the Royal College of Nursing has published an excellent booklet for nursing students about bullying and harassment.

REFERENCES

NMC 2002a Guidelines for the administration of medicines. NMC, London
NMC 2002b Guidelines for records and record keeping. NMC, London

Appendix 11.1: NMC *Guidelines for Records and Record Keeping*

Foreword

The Nursing and Midwifery Council [NMC] believes that record keeping is a fundamental part of nursing and midwifery practice. As the regulatory body for these professions, we have a legal responsibility to provide advice to registered nurses and midwives on standards of professional practice. In 1993, the former United Kingdom Central Council for Nursing, Midwifery and Health Visiting [UKCC] published the first edition of *Standards for Records* and record keeping in order to give guidance in this area to registrants. The UKCC published a revised second edition of the publication, entitled *Guidelines for Records and Record Keeping*, in 1998. This NMC advisory booklet is simply a reprint of the 1998 publication.

The guidance is based upon extensive consultation with organizations representing the interests of patients and clients, registered nurses and midwives, professional organizations and trades unions, employers, managers and legal experts in record keeping. The consultation included conferences, individual submissions and discussions, together with comments upon an earlier draft of the text.

Like all NMC guidance, this is not a rule book that will provide the answer to every question or issue that could ever arise in the area of record keeping. Nor do we believe that it is the role of the NMC in this respect to define a rigid framework for the content and format of your record keeping. Instead, we seek to provide guidelines that we hope will help you to think through some of the issues and to exercise your professional judgement as an individual accountable registered nurse or midwife. We hope that you will find this booklet helpful to you in all aspects of your professional practice.

Introduction

Record keeping is an integral part of nursing and midwifery practice. It is a tool of professional practice and one that should help the care process. It is not separate from this process and it is not an optional extra to be fitted in if circumstances allow.

Good record keeping helps to protect the welfare of patients and clients by promoting:

- high standards of clinical care
- continuity of care
- better communication and dissemination of information between members of the inter-professional health care team
- an accurate account of treatment and care planning and delivery
- the ability to detect problems, such as changes in the patient's or client's condition, at an early stage.

The quality of your record keeping is also a reflection of the standard of your professional practice. Good record keeping is a mark of the skilled and safe practitioner, whilst careless or incomplete record keeping often highlights wider problems with the individual's practice.

There is no single model or template for a record. The best record is one that is the product of the consultation and discussion which has taken place at a local level between all members of the inter-professional health care team and the patient or client. It is one that is evaluated and adapted in response to the needs of patients and clients. It is one that enables any registrant to care for the patient or client, regardless of where they are within the care process or care environment. It is an invaluable way of promoting communication within the health care team and between practitioners and their patients or clients. Good record keeping is, therefore, both the product of good team work and an important tool in promoting high quality health care.

The NMC believes that there are a number of key principles that underpin good records and record keeping. Some of these relate to the content and style of the record. In addition, there are some legal issues that you, as a registered nurse or midwife, should be aware of and take into account in your record keeping practice.

The following sections set out these principles and legal aspects. They are designed to help you to reflect upon your current record keeping practice and how you can develop it in order to benefit your patients and clients.

The principles set out in this document apply across all care settings and to both manual and computer-held records. The NMC accepts that, until there is national agreement between all health care professions on standards and format, records may differ depending on the needs of the patient or client. The record must, however, follow a logical and methodical sequence with clear milestones and goals for the record keeping process.

Content and style

There are a number of factors that contribute to effective record keeping. Patient and client records should:

- be factual, consistent and accurate
- be written as soon as possible after an event has occurred, providing current information on the care and condition of the patient or client
- be written clearly and in such a manner that the text cannot be erased
- be written in such a manner that any alterations or additions are dated, timed and signed in such a way that the original entry can still be read clearly
- be accurately dated, timed and signed, with the signature printed alongside the first entry
- not include abbreviations, jargon, meaningless phrases, irrelevant speculation and offensive subjective statements
- be readable on any photocopies.

In addition, records should:

- be written, wherever possible, with the involvement of the patient, client or their carer
- be written in terms that the patient or client can understand

- be consecutive
- identify problems that have arisen and the action taken to rectify them
- provide clear evidence of the care planned, the decisions made, the care delivered and the information shared.

Audit

Audit is one component of the risk management process, the aim of which is the promotion of quality. If improvements are identified and made in the processes and outcomes of health care, risks to the patient or client are minimized and costs to the employer are reduced.

Audit can play a vital part in ensuring the quality of care that is delivered and this applies equally to the process of record keeping. By auditing your records, you can assess the standard of the records and identify areas for improvement and staff development. Audit tools should therefore be devised at a local level to monitor the standard of the records produced and to form a basis both for discussion and measurement. Whatever audit tool or system is used, it should primarily be directed towards serving the interests of your patients and clients, rather than organizational convenience. You may also wish to consider including a system of peer review in the process. The need to maintain confidentiality of patient and client information applies to audit just as to the record keeping process itself.

Legal matters and complaints

Patient and client records are sometimes called in evidence before a court of law, by the Health Service Commissioner or in order to investigate a complaint at a local level. They may also be used in evidence by the NMC's Professional Conduct Committee, which considers complaints about professional misconduct by registered nurses and midwives. Care plans, diaries, birth plans and anything that makes reference to the care of the patient or client may be required as evidence.

As a registered nurse or midwife, you have both a professional and a legal duty of care. Your record keeping should therefore be able to demonstrate:

- a full account of your assessment and the care you have planned and provided
- relevant information about the condition of the patient or client at any given time and the measures you have taken to respond to their needs
- evidence that you have understood and honoured your duty of care, that you have taken all reasonable steps to care for the patient or client and that any actions or omissions on your part have not compromised their safety in any way
- a record of any arrangements you have made for the continuing care of a patient or client.

The frequency of entries will be determined both by your professional judgement and local standards and agreements. You will need to exercise particular care and make more frequent entries when patients or clients present complex problems, show deviation from the norm, require more intensive care than normal, are confused and disoriented or generally give cause for concern. You must use your professional judgement (if necessary in discussion with other members of the health care team) to determine when these circumstances exist.

The approach to record keeping that courts of law adopt tends to be that 'if it is not recorded, it has not been done'. You must use your professional judgement to decide what is relevant and what should be recorded. This applies particularly to situations where the condition of the patient or client is apparently unchanging and no record has been made of the care delivered. Local standards should be set to define what is a reasonable time lapse if this is the case. Midwives must ensure that they are aware of and comply with the requirements set out in the NMC's *Midwives Rules and Code of Practice* that relate to the maintenance and retention of records.

If you are working with clients who are subject to mental health legislation, you must ensure that you have a thorough working knowledge of these statutory powers as they apply to your particular area of practice. When making entries in records for these clients, you must comply as appropriate with the guidance given by the Mental Health Act Commission for England and Wales, the Mental Welfare Commission for Scotland or the Mental Health Commission for Northern Ireland.

In making a record, you should also be aware of the reliance which your professional colleagues will have upon it. Good communication is therefore essential. Furthermore, you are professionally accountable for ensuring that any duties that you delegate to those members of the inter-professional health care team who are not registered practitioners are undertaken to a reasonable standard.

For instance, if you delegate record keeping to pre-registration students of nursing or midwifery or to health care assistants, you must ensure that they are adequately supervised and that they are competent to perform the task. You must clearly countersign any such entry and remember that you are professionally accountable for the consequences of such an entry. You must ensure that any entry you make in a record can easily be identified. If your signature is unclear, you should print your name alongside it. You are strongly advised not to use your initials only as a signature.

Access and ownership

You need to assume that any entries you make in a patient or client record will be scrutinized at some point. Patients and clients not only have a legal right to see their records but they are increasingly participating in writing and holding them.

Access to records – legal aspects

The *Access to Health Records Act 1990* gives patients and clients the right of access to manual health records about themselves that were made after 1 November 1991.

The *Data Protection Act 1984* gives patients and clients access to their computer-held records. It also regulates the storage and protection of patient and client information held on computer.

In some cases, registered nurses and midwives can withhold information from a patient or client that they believe could cause serious harm to the physical or mental health of the patient or client, or which would breach the confidentiality of another patient or client. If you make the decision to withhold information in this way, you must be able to justify it and you must record it. The system for dealing with applications for access is explained in the *Guide to the Access to Health Records Act 1990*, which is published by the government health departments. As a registered nurse or midwife, you must be aware of the rights of patients or clients in these circumstances.

Inter-professional access to records

The NMC supports the principle of shared records in which all members of the health care team involved in the care and treatment of an individual make entries in a single record and in accordance with an agreed local protocol. The ability to obtain information whilst respecting patient and client confidentiality is essential. Each practitioner's contribution to such records should be seen as of equal importance. This reflects the wider value of collaborative working within the inter-professional health care team.

The same right of access to records by the patient or client exists where a system of shared records is in use. It is essential, therefore, that local agreement is reached to identify and publicize who is responsible for considering requests from patients and clients for access in particular circumstances.

Retention

The period for which patient or client records may be required to be kept can depend upon a number of pieces of legislation or health services policy statements issued by government health departments. Your employer should have protocols that you should follow and which will probably require you to keep any record you have made for at least eight years and, in the case of a child, at least to the date of the child's 21st birthday. If you are self-employed, you should also ensure that no record you have made relating to the care of a patient or client is destroyed within a period of eight, or 21, years respectively as above.

Ownership of records

Organizations that employ professional staff who make records are the legal owners of those records. This does not mean, however, that anyone in the organization has an automatic right of access to the records or the information contained within them. You have a duty to protect the confidentiality of the patient or client record. This is particularly important when there are potential areas of conflict, such as occupational health records, where the record itself belongs to the organization but the information contained in the record is confidential and should only be released, even to someone within the organization, with the consent of the patient or client.

Patient-held records

Patients and clients increasingly own their health care records and this should be encouraged as far as it is appropriate and as long as they are happy to do so. It enables them to be more closely involved in their own care and enables you to share with them the information that you consider relevant to your assessment and care of them. Patients and clients should be informed of the purpose and importance of the record and their responsibility for keeping it safe. These same principles apply equally to parent-held records.

Sometimes, you may feel that your particular concerns or anxieties require you to keep a supplementary record to which access by the patient, client or family members is limited or withheld. Keeping a supplementary record should be the exception rather than the norm, however, and should not extend to keeping full duplicate records. Wherever possible, concerns should be shared with the patient or client and the relevant entry should be jointly compiled. You must be able to justify keeping such a supplementary record and its existence needs to be made clear to other members of the health care team, who must be able to access the information readily but without compromising patient and client confidentiality.

Research, teaching and access

Patient and client records may be used for research, teaching purposes and clinical supervision. The principles of access and confidentiality remain the same and the right of the patient or client to refuse access to their records should be respected. The use of patient or client records in research should be approved by your local research ethics committee.

Information technology and computer-held records

Many registered nurses and midwives are now regularly using information technology to record the planning, assessment and delivery of care. There are obvious advantages to this. Computer-held records tend to be easier to read, less bulky, reduce the need for duplication and can increase communication across the inter-professional health care team. However, the same basic principles that apply to manual records must be applied to computer-held records. You do not need to keep manual duplicates of computer-held records and they do not replace the need to maintain dialogue throughout the inter-professional health care team.

Security, access and confidentiality

The principle of the confidentiality of information held about your patients and clients is just as important in computer-held records as in all other records, including those sent by fax. You are professionally accountable for making sure that whatever system is used is fully secure. Clear local protocols should be drawn up to specify which staff have access to computer-held records. Although patients and clients can expect their health records to be accessed by different members of the inter-professional health care team, this should only be done where necessary.

Patients and clients do not have the right to limit the amount of information relevant to their care or condition that is incorporated in their records. However, they can limit access to certain information about themselves and you must respect their right to do so. Local guidelines and protocols should address this right and these procedures should also include ways of establishing the date and time of any entry, the person who made the entry, and should ensure that any changes or additions to entries are made in such a way that the original information is still visible and accessible.

Patient and client involvement

As with manual records, patients and clients should be equal partners, whenever possible, in the compilation of their own records. The *Data Protection Act 1984*, the *Access Modification (Health) Order 1987*, the *Access to Health Records Act 1990* and the *Access to Health Records (Northern Ireland) Order 1993* define their rights of access.

Accountability and computer-held records

You are accountable for any entry you make to a computer-held record and you must ensure that any entry you make is clearly identifiable.

Further information and advice

We hope that you have found this booklet helpful. Further information and advice are available by contacting the NMC's professional advice service by telephone on 020 7333 6541/6550/6553, by e-mail at advice@nmc-uk.org, by fax on 020 7333 6538 or via the NMC's website at www.nmc-uk.org. For a list of current NMC publications, please refer to our website at www.nmc-uk.org or write to the Publications Department at the NMC's address or by e-mail at publications@nmc-uk.org.

Please note that copies of the government legislation cited in these guidelines are available from your local branch of The Stationery Office and not from the NMC.

Published by the former United Kingdom Central Council for Nursing, Midwifery and Health Visiting in October 1998. Reprinted by the Nursing and Midwifery Council in April 2002.

Reproduced with permission of the NMC.

Summary

- Record keeping is an integral part of nursing and midwifery practice.

- Good record keeping is a mark of the skilled and safe practitioner.

- Records should not include abbreviations, jargon, meaningless phrases, irrelevant speculation and offensive subjective statements.

- Records should be written in terms that the patient or client can easily understand.

- By auditing your records, you can assess the standard of the record and identify areas for improvement and staff development.

- You must ensure that any entry you make in a record can easily be identified.

- Patients and clients have the right of access to records held about them.

- Each practitioner's contribution to records should be seen as of equal importance.

- You have a duty to protect the confidentiality of the patient and client record.

- Patients and clients should own their health care records as far as it is appropriate and as long as they are happy to do so.

- The principle of the confidentiality of information held about your patients and clients is just as important in computer-held records as in all other records.

- The use of records in research should be approved by your local research ethics committee.

- You must use your professional judgement to decide what is relevant and what should be recorded.

- Records should be written clearly and in such a manner that the text can not be erased.
- Records should be factual, consistent and accurate.
- You need to assume that any entries you make in a patient or client record will be scrutinized at some point.
- Good record keeping helps to protect the welfare of patients and clients.

Final Thoughts

First, I want to thank you for reading this book; I hope that it has helped and encouraged you to stay with your course and to become a nurse. Those are really the only reasons it was written – to make your course easier and to help you become a better nurse.

When I started to write it, I realized that I had been through the stress of a pre-registration nursing course twice – once in the UK and once in America. For some reason, I thought that qualified me to write this book.

As much as this book has (I hope) been a voyage of discovery to read, it has also been a voyage of discovery for me to write it. I have had to look even more closely at my own skills and knowledge as I tried to pass some of them on to you. While writing this, I was also completing my District Nursing course so I was a student, too!

I have tried to explain things as if you were my own student and I was your mentor. And even though I don't know you by name, I feel like I know who you are. And I hope this book has shown you that I care – and most of the nurses out here are like me. We just don't always show it because there are so many things going on, but we *are* glad to have you. And I would like to apologize for us all in advance for those times when you need us to show you we understand but we are too busy to notice. The men and women who have become nurses are a good group of people and we really are looking forward to you joining us. But, you have to survive your course first.

Your success depends not on your academic ability, your experience in health care, or even on your overall 'nursiness'. Those who finish the course do it because they were the ones who didn't give up. That's why I want to give you these final thoughts:

❜ Nothing in the world can take the place of persistence. Talent will not; nothing is more common than unsuccessful men with

talent. Genius will not; unrewarded genius is almost a proverb. Education will not; the world is full of educated derelicts. Persistence and determination are omnipotent. The slogan 'press on' has solved and will solve the problems of the human race.
(Calvin Coolidge, 30th President of the United States of America)

And that's where I leave you – press on. Some days you will want to hide and cry, others you will just wish you could stay in bed. You will have sleepless nights and stress-filled weekends. But I promise that the good will outweigh the bad and you will be through the course before you know it. Just keep putting one foot in front of the other.

Don't give up on yourself. Be patient with friends and family who are struggling to get through your course almost as much as you are! Lean on your friends in the course and let them know they can lean on you. Say thank you to mentors and tutors who really make a difference so you can encourage them to keep working so hard. Don't let a bad grade or a bad experience knock your confidence. Don't hide it when you need help, and don't be silent when you should speak up for yourself.

Know that you can do it. Press on!

Bethann

Useful Books, Journals and Other Resources

SUGGESTED BOOKS AND RESOURCES

I have read or used each of these books, either in the current or an older edition. I have hundreds of nursing books; I have recommended those I believe will help you the most. But before you buy a book, look at it in the library and try to decide if the value the book will give you is worth the cover price. Some are worth buying, others are more useful if you just borrow them occasionally.

I believe that most of the books I have listed here are worth buying (feel free to copy this and send it out as a Christmas or birthday list) because you will get your money out of them as a student or you will be able to use them as a nurse as well.

I prefer to buy my books new, so I can take care of them and keep them in good shape but you can buy books second hand, sometimes at your uni but also from eBay (www.ebay.com) and Amazon (www.amazon.co.uk). Be aware that second-hand books might not be the most current edition and might not be in great shape.

A note about web sites – they go out of date very quickly, so I haven't put many here. There are hundreds of useful sites; when you find a good one, share it with your colleagues.

Finally, I haven't referred to books that are specific to four Branches. You will have time during your common foundation programme to find out which books are most useful – through your lecturers, library and students who are ahead of you in the Branch.

Bullying

www.bullyonline.org/

> *This website is funny, informative and very direct. If you are dealing with a bully or just want to know more, go to this website. It's brilliant and very useful.*

Clinical skills

Jamieson E, McCall J, Whyte E 2002 Clinical nursing practices. Churchill Livingstone, Edinburgh

A good basic book that explains the procedures every nurse needs to know from basics like how to take a temperature to more complicated procedures like how to assist at a liver biopsy. Reflects on the activities of living categories for each procedure. It is a 'must' for a new student who is inexperienced in healthcare and is also useful for more experienced students who are transitioning from an HCA to a nursing role.

Skinner S 1998 Understanding drug therapies. Baillière Tindall, London

A good book to help you understand different drug classes and how they act. Easy to read but thorough.

Walsh M, Ford P 1989 Nursing rituals, research and rational actions. Heinemann, Oxford

An old book that you can get used from eBay or Amazon. I found it very enlightening and useful. It discusses the reasons we do things as nurses. It's written in a personable and enjoyable way.

Mallett J, Dougherty L 2000 The Royal Marsden hospital manual of clinical nursing procedures, 5th edn. Blackwell, Oxford

Also simply called 'The Marsden Manual'. It gives step-by-step outlines, including rationales and explanations, for most nursing procedures. It is a definitive guide to clinical practice and although not cheap, is a good investment.

Common foundation programme

Kenworthy N, Snowley G, Gilling C (eds) 2002 Common foundation studies in nursing, 3rd edn. Churchill Livingstone, Edinburgh

Great book, offers in-depth information about essential topics. Will guide you through your common foundation programme.

Heath H (ed) 1995 Potter and Perry's foundations in nursing theory and practice. Mosby, London

An all-round basic text, with information relevant to all four Branches. It covers basic concepts like 'what is nursing' through to medications and wound care. An excellent, but old, text. I can't find any newer edition than this 1995 one, a factor that is seriously against this book.

However, it is still an excellent resource, although if you can only afford one, buy the Kenworthy one above.

Ethics

Rumbold G 2000 Ethics in nursing practice, 3rd edn. Baillière Tindall, Edinburgh
    Easy to read, presented plainly and in clear language. Discusses relationships with patients and other professionals, and the way ethics impact on decisions nurses make. A classic book and a real 'must have'.

Health promotion

Naidoo J, Wills J 2000 Health promotion, 2nd edn. Baillière Tindall, London
    An excellent basic health promotion text. Outlines everything from how to assess a community's health to strategies to improve health and evaluate the effectiveness of those strategies. Clear and plainly written. Useful in community nursing modules.

Leadership

www.nwlink.com/~donclark/leader/leader.html
    This is a great site with a lot of information, links and it is all presented in a clear, easy to understand but comprehensive manner.
www.nursingleadership.co.uk
    Government nurse leadership project homepage.

Learning styles

Hinchliff S, Eaton A, Howard S, Thompson S 2003 Practitioner as teacher, 3rd edn. Churchill Livingstone, Edinburgh
    This book is really intended for qualified nurses who want to be a mentor or teacher, but it's a good resource for a student nurse too. It discusses the way people learn and learning in the clinical environment. Light, clear and easy to read. Lets you in on what your mentors and teachers are trying to do!

Legal issues

Dimond B 2001 Legal aspects of nursing, 3rd edn. Prentice-Hall, London
    I don't know this book well but it comes very highly recommended as the best general book about legal issues in nursing.

Models and theories

If you become very interested in a specific model, you can look for additional information by that specific nursing theorist in your library.

Pearson A, Vaughn B, Fitzgerald M 1996 Nursing models for practice, 2nd edn. Butterworth-Heinemann, Oxford
> *Easy to read and understand, very clear and although not really comprehensive should give you anything that you need.*

Nursing practice

Hinchliff S, Norman S, Schober J 2003 Nursing practice and health care: a foundation text, 4th edn. Arnold, London
> *A clearly written book that explains elements of care in common foundation and in each of the different Branches. It is great for helping you learn to think and behave as a nurse. An excellent resource for assignments as well.*

Walsh M (ed) 2002 Watson's clinical nursing and related sciences, 6th edn. Baillière Tindall, Edinburgh
> *Approaches patient care system by system. Is comprehensive but easy to read. A good investment as it discusses not only the nursing care but also the related anatomy and physiology. Great to use for preparing for placements and will be useful after your course.*

Research

Craig J, Smyth R 2002 The evidence-based practice manual for nurses. Churchill Livingstone, Edinburgh
> *Most of this is a little advanced for a brand new student but it has an absolutely brilliant section on how to do a literature search. Worth buying just for that chapter. Has an impressive list of resources to help you search.*

Lanoe N 2002 Ogier's reading research: how to make research more approachable, 3rd edn. Baillière Tindall, London
> *Good book that will guide you through reading and thinking about research, although it won't really help you write research.*

Parahoo K 1997 Nursing research: principles, process and issues. Palgrave, Basingstoke
> *A great book that can help you understand or actually do research. Clearly written with good examples and explanations.*

Reflection

There is a lot available online and in journals about reflection, and reflection is mentioned in nursing texts about many other subjects. The Maslin-Prothero book in the study skills section is very good on reflection. If you do decide to buy a book, look at the two below, or find something that you can relate to by looking at reflective practice books in the nursing library before buying one.

Johns C 2000 Becoming a reflective practitioner: a reflective and holistic approach to clinical nursing, practice development and clinical supervision. Blackwell Science, Oxford

Johns C, Freshwater D (eds) 1998 Transforming nursing through reflective practice. Blackwell Science, Oxford

Social policy

Although a good book can help you understand the background to current policy, social policy changes faster than any textbook can follow. For the most current things, look at the Department of Health and NHS websites (always read the executive summary before wading through any government document).

Ham C 1999 Health policy in Britain: the politics and organization of the National Health Service, 4th edn. Palgrave, Basingstoke
> *This book is pretty easy to read, considering the subject matter, and helps you understand not just about where policy has come from, but why it evolved the way it did.*

www.doh.gov.uk
www.nhs.uk
You can look at national sites as well.
www.show.scot.nhs.uk/index.aspx
www.scotland.gov.uk/who/dept_health.asp
www.wales.gov.uk/subihealth/index.htm
www.wales.nhs.uk/
www.dhsspsni.gov.uk/
www.n-i.nhs.uk/

Study skills

Goodall C 1995 A survivor's guide to study skills and student assessments. Churchill Livingstone, Edinburgh
> *A basic book, light to read but very useful.*

Maslin-Prothero Sian (ed) 2001 Baillière's study skills for nurses, 2nd edn. Baillière Tindall, London
> *A good basic all-round book, very thorough and easy to read. If you only get one study skills book, get this one.*

Taylor J 1992 Study skills for nurses. Chapman Hall, London
> *A small, older book but has good hints and tips about presentations and seminars among other things.*

MAGAZINES AND JOURNALS

For CFP students, the *Nursing Standard* (*NS*) and the *Nursing Times* (*NT*) are great reading and have special rates for students. You can also access them online through your uni's library resources. These are great gifts to ask your family for. Search for 'Nursing Standard' or 'Nursing Times' online to access their home pages. If you buy one copy (which they will have in your uni's shop or at any hospital newsagent) there is information inside on how to subscribe.

There are other journals. *British Journal of Nursing* (*BJN*) is great but might be a little advanced for a new student. Wait until you are at the end of your second or beginning of your third year to get this journal to make sure you are up to it.

The publishers of the *NS*, *NT* and *BJN* put out some specialty journals. You might be able to get a discount but this is not offered on all of them.

There are many nursing magazines from the US but be careful, because standards of practice and care systems are very different and the material might not fit in with your role as a nurse in the UK.

The National Union of Students (NUS)

You might encounter two types of 'student union' while you are a student. There is the National Union of Students (NUS) – an organization that supports students in many different capacities across the UK (there are NUS branches in each of the four UK countries) – or unions of students that are not affiliated with the NUS. Even if your local office is not specifically affiliated with the NUS, it will still offer support and help. You can get a lot of information about the NUS quite easily:

- Pop into the NUS office on your campus (the best way).
- Go to www.nusonline.co.uk (the next best way).
- Call your university switchboard and ask to speak to the union of students office (from personal experience, some receptionists will not be very well informed or will be very busy – it's better to go in person or check the web!).

What does the NUS offer you?

- Your NUS card, which entitles you to many different student discounts and which is accepted as proof of your student status in most places.
- Information about benefits and discounts for students.
- Support for international students.
- Help with government forms such as entitlement to free prescriptions.
- Documents about student issues such as housing and finances.
- Publications about every aspect of university and student life.
- Advice from advisors trained to support students who are having academic, personal or financial problems.
- Help in planning events like a student ball or other student activity.

- Help in joining a union or any student group/organization.
- The NUS usually runs a shop for students, and often runs a bar as well.
- Activities and fun events on campus.
- Representation in academic (but not clinical placement related) disciplinary proceedings and cheating boards.
- A university newsletter or newspaper.
- Fresher's fayres.
- Advocacy for national student issues – the NUS sends representatives to political party conferences, meets with governmental officials, and has advisors and elected officials working actively to promote student welfare through government support and policy.

In addition, if you are a group rep, or steward/representative for Unison, the Royal College of Nursing or the Royal College of Midwives, the NUS office can often offer you some office space and support for official duties.

Your university gives the NUS funding based on student numbers (it's usually a pound or less per head). Sadly, some campuses or satellites that have mainly or all nursing students have a history of not being as well supported as the campuses that have 'traditional' students (you know, the recent school leavers who attend classes Monday to Friday, 9 a.m. to 3.30 p.m. and who have regular holidays and the summer off) – if you need help, speak up. The NUS is usually very good at adapting to meeting students needs. You can also run for local, regional or national office in the NUS!

In addition to supporting students, the NUS represents the student viewpoint by organizing and participating in demonstrations, lobbying government and raising money for local and national charities.

However, there are a few problems for the NUS in helping nursing students: First, the influx of large numbers of nursing students has perhaps overwhelmed the NUS a bit; second, the emergence of satellite campuses devoted to nursing but without (usually) student residences and without university offices (the usual locations for NUS offices); and third, the schedules for nursing courses (throughout the summer, in the evening and even some weekends) have made it difficult for the NUS to keep up with the demand for services. At this time, the NUS doesn't have the resources or information to help student nurses with problems related specifically to clinical placements. However, it has identified many of these issues as problems that must be addressed and is trying to put in place national level representatives whose role it is to look into and support the types of problems student nurses have – both as a result of their course and in accessing NUS services.

What should you go to the NUS for? (not all NUS offices will offer everything – if you need something, just call or drop in and ask):

- **Academic problems:** when you think something is unfair, when you think the university has violated a policy or correct procedure, when you have been accused of an academic offence like cheating, or when you need help with academic skills. The NUS will also support your group reps (students elected in each cohort to represent student perspectives on university governance groups and to raise concerns and issues).
- **Complaints:** you can raise complaints and concerns about the university, campus, university housing, etc. through the NUS.
- **Personal problems:** relationship problems, health issues, bullying, mental health, issues related to sexuality and sexual health, financial problems, disabilities, problems or questions about housing, etc. They also offer advice on crime prevention and safety. You can usually get an inexpensive personal alarm through the NUS.
- **Lifestyle:** information about discounts, the local nightlife, events, student-friendly businesses, part-time work, support for international students, etc. The NUS has career information (not a lot of it is great for nurses, but they are improving this), and can give advice and guidance about CVs and interviews.
- **Activities:** the NUS office will have information on clubs, sports, organizations and groups on campus. They also will

support you if you want to plan a trip, event, or activitiy such as a graduation ball (hint: you need at least a year to plan a graduation ball, in part because of placements but also because it takes a lot of time – go see them sooner rather than later!).

- **Other resources:** The NUS will be able to point you in the direction of someone who can help you if they can't. They will have many valuable publications from the NUS, from the university, and from other organizations.
- Fax and photocopy services.

The NUS is an excellent organization that offers support and assistance in nearly every type of query or problem you may have. **It does *not*, however, offer any support or assistance if your problem is related to clinical placements.** You are still likely to need help and support from one of the unions that support nursing students (Unison, the Royal College of Nursing or the Royal College of Midwives). Each of these organizations has special resources and information targeted specifically for nursing (or midwifery) students.

Go and visit your student union office; get your NUS card; see what's on offer and if you have a little time or some expertise in a particular area – offer to help. The NUS is for students, by students … it can always use your help and support.

Tips for Mental Health Student Nurses

1. Remember that mental health impacts on physical health, and physical health impacts on mental health.

2. Just because someone is mentally ill doesn't mean that they can't give (or deny) consent. Most people with mental illness lead independent lives and are able to make good decisions for themselves.

3. Never ever be untruthful. Once you have lost trust, you have nothing to work with. Never tell a client that you will keep a secret. You can't help them if you aren't honest.

4. There's a saying: 'Just because you're paranoid doesn't mean that someone isn't out to get you!' Remember that no matter what a person's illness is, you still must take their complaints seriously. Don't just assume that someone complaining of pain or other symptoms is exhibiting attention-seeking behaviour.

5. Good boundaries are essential. You need to be aware of emotional and physical boundaries; someone with a mental illness may misinterpret actions or comments you make. Be careful so you can continue to be therapeutic for your clients. Don't dress in a way that could upset your clients: football strips, clothes with logos or political/religious symbols or that could be considered revealing/provocative could all upset clients with mental illness. Dress in a neutral, professional way. Also be aware as well that some clients could react to your size, colour, shape, hair colour, body jewellery, tattoos, etc.

6. Some people with mental illness can be very manipulative or charismatic. Be cautious and always be objective. Always leave yourself a way out of a situation – never allow a client to get between you and an exit. You can't help people if you don't keep yourself safe.

7. Some people will never get any better, and for some people what appear to be insignificant achievements are major triumphs. Praise your clients for their hard work.

8. As a student, you should *never* provide one-to-one supervision for a client. You yourself need supervision, so how can you supervise anyone else?

9. A person is not their diagnosis. Just because there are many common characteristics in a disease doesn't mean any person is a 'typical manic' or a 'typical schizophrenic'. See your clients as individuals and don't fall into the habit of seeing people only as their disease.

10. Many nurses in all different Branches and areas suffer from stress and stress-related problems. Don't try to cure yourself through your job. You are there to be therapeutic for your clients, not for them to help you.

Learning Disability Nursing

Denise Stevens

One of the first things I wanted to learn as a student nurse in learning disability nursing was: what do qualified nurses actually do? I was several months into my nurse training at university before my first practical placement and I actually had no idea of what nurses in this field did. I very excitedly asked my fellow students who had previously worked as support staff in residential homes for adults with learning disabilities, only to discover that everyone appeared to have their own ideas of what constituted an RNLD. One student even suggested that learning disability nurses spent their days travelling around weighing clients!

HISTORY

The historical 'care' or 'treatment' of learning disabled people has had an enormous impact on the current role of the RNLD. For example, as long ago as the fifteenth century, people with a learning disability were stigmatized and considered to be lunatics. Treatment consisted of being chained and whipped (Gates 1997). In the sixteenth century, learning disabilities were linked to witchcraft and learning disabled people were locked away, often with keepers they feared. In the eighteenth and nineteenth centuries those considered to be 'lunatics' were separated from paupers. Aristocratic patients often lived in private asylums that provided accommodation of a similar level of comfort to that found in upper-class family homes (Scull 1979) but, despite the surroundings, few improved and the private asylums were in fact just luxurious prisons. In comparison, the private madhouses that housed pauper 'lunatics' were described as desperately cruel and conditions were abominable (Scull, 1979). Treatment consisted of bleeding, digitalis, electricity and emetics (Gates 1997). Many patients were kept in irons; there were no baths, books, employment and often only one staff member to as many as 50 patients. Reforms brought in the nineteenth century were initially intended to cure patients but with the low cure rates the emphasis changed to providing more humane living conditions, such as clean bedding, sufficient clothing, an absence of chains and regular attendance at church.

In the mid-twentieth century, Nazi Germany exterminated people with a mental handicap, along with others they considered to be undesirable.

It was not until the 1970s that conditions for people with learning disabilities finally began to improve, after damaging publicity regarding the ill treatment and substandard living conditions in large institutions. Patients often had no personal possessions, clothing or space (Swann 1997). Barton (1960) identified a separate condition known as 'institutional neurosis', which resulted from the institutionalized care received by people with learning disabilities in mental hospitals. The condition was characterized by apathy, lack of initiative or interest, submissiveness, deterioration in personal habits and resignation to their surroundings. The White Paper *Better Services for the Mentally Handicapped* was published in 1971 but it was not until 1990 that the NHS and Community Care Act became law.

THE PRESENT DAY

The implementation of the 1990 Act was the beginning of the slow move from institutional care to improved community care. The care of people with learning disabilities has evolved over centuries, with the most dramatic changes occurring since the 1970s with the concept of deinstitutionalization and normalization.

The concept of normalization was developed as long ago as 1959 in Denmark and 1969 in Sweden (Swann 1997).

Wolfensberger (1972) states that normalization seeks to value client groups who were previously devalued. To do this, Wolfensberger (1972) promoted social role valorization and believed that people with learning disabilities needed to be seen to be leading socially valued lives by living as part of the community, accessing local facilities and having the same rights and opportunities as everyone else. Many trusts now use the John O'Brien five service accomplishments as a method of implementing the concept of normalization into care delivery. This is considered to be a 'user friendly' approach that gives a set of values together with a framework for use (Plougher 1997).

It is these basic philosophies of normalization and social role valorization that underpin the work of the nurse in learning disabilities and service provision. In response to the considerable changes in the care of people with learning disabilities and deinstitutionalization, the role of the nurse in learning disabilities has also had to adapt and evolve, and is continuing to do so.

Fortunately, the role of the nurse in learning disabilities is no longer deciding which chains to use, and working in this service is now extremely rewarding. It is now possible to play an important role in facilitating people to be as independent as possible and to have real choices over their own lives.

THE ROLE OF THE LEARNING DISABILITY NURSE

There would appear to be many views on the role of the learning disabilities nurse. According to Baldwin and Birchenall (Gates 1997) there are six key roles: clinician, counsellor, advisor/advocate, manager, educator and therapist. As with all branches of nursing, the nursing intervention depends on the needs of the individual. For example, a person with a mild learning disability may be able to live independently, be in employment and only need nursing intervention for reasons such as administration of medication, dietary advice or monitoring. A person with a profound learning disability may also be physically disabled with no sensory, communication or learning ability and be completely dependent on carers for all of their personal and health needs. There are also some people with learning disabilities who present with severe behavioural problems that require specialist knowledge and skills. These behaviours can also vary, from people with poor social skills or inappropriate sexual behaviour, to those who exhibit aggressive, threatening or self-injurious behaviour. There are also learning disability nurses working in the forensic service with offenders, for example sex offenders and fire setters. These varied roles are unique to the RNLD. According to Butler (2003) skills such as 'high level social development and behavioural knowledge' (p. 28) are what make learning disability nurses so highly valued. It must also be remembered that people with learning disabilities have the same health problems as the rest of society, as well as the unique health issues of those with genetic disorders and syndromes.

Life in learning disability nursing can also be extremely interesting, providing the setting for many anecdotal stories. For example …

On one occasion a young, male client was staring quite intently. When asked if he was all right he shook his head to indicate that he was not. He was asked if he wanted something to which he nodded his head to indicate 'yes'. When asked what he would like his answer can only be described as 'personal services'! I had to explain to him that this was not in my remit as a student nurse, I was unable to oblige and he was offered a cup of tea instead!

Always read client care plans

Because of the very diverse client groups within the learning disability service, each with their unique needs, the 'top tips' to students are also very client specific. However, there is some advice that may be useful to all student nurses in learning disabilities. For example, always read client care plans as soon as possible when on placement. There may be clients who exhibit challenging behaviours and have behavioural programmes in place. The care plans will give information as to triggers to the behaviours and advice on how to manage them. It is only when everyone who is involved with the client works consistently that behavioural programmes can be successful in reducing unwanted behaviours. It can take only one person to seriously undermine and jeopardize success. Reading client care plans will inform you of any client allergies, preferences or dislikes. An example of this is that many learning disabled adults have been subject to abuse: whether physical, sexual, psychological or financial. A client who has suffered previous abuse may not like a particular gender to be involved in his or her personal care. He or she may not like physical touch and will react quite strongly when touched, even accidentally. It is also important to remember that any new face on a unit, even a well-intentioned student, can be very unsettling for a person with a learning disability. It can take time to earn the trust and confidence of a client, so taking the time to get to know someone before being involved in their personal care is good practice.

Always read trust policies

It is also important to read local trust policies and procedures, together with any specific unit policies. It is important for student nurses to work in accordance with trust policies. It cannot be assumed that all staff work in accordance to these policies but by being informed of expected practices a student nurse can avoid being compromised.

BEING A STUDENT NURSE

Every student nurse should be aware of the Nursing and Midwifery Council (NMC) guidelines for student nurses. Students are sometimes asked to carry out duties that are inappropriate and unacceptable, and this can seriously risk patient safety. For example: one first-year student nurse on her first practical placement was asked to fit a male catheter, and although this was by a very insistent doctor, she had the good sense to refuse; a second-year student nurse was asked to administer client medication in a nursing home environment without the supervision of qualified or drug assessed staff and she was encouraged to take sole responsibility for this duty. Drug errors are all too easy to make for even the most diligent of qualified nurses, and can be potentially fatal, so it is understandable that the administration of medicines by unsupervised student nurses is against all guidelines and policies. Medication charts in learning disability premises often have an accompanying photograph of the client to aid recognition – extremely useful when being asked to administer medication in an unfamiliar environment.

The open culture in nursing now encourages disclosure of mistakes as a learning tool for others. A nurse is no longer disciplined for medication errors but will be disciplined for not following procedure. If an error occurs, be honest and ensure the correct care for the client, do not try to cover it up because it is professional suicide and clearly not in the client's best interest. Several fellow students have been asked to lift clients physically – without the use of hoisting equipment – this was accepted practice by regular staff despite there being 'no lifting' policies. The students felt isolated when taking a stand against lifting clients but nurses and student nurses alike need to advocate good, safe, legal practice. Also, if a student nurse is injured when physically lifting a client he or she will not be insured!

Occasional 'pockets' of staff do not adhere to the philosophy of normalization and do not work with learning disabled clients in a respectful or dignified way. It can be difficult for a student nurse to flag up problem areas or concerns when on practical placement, and he or she may have difficult choices to make, especially given the need to pass placements. But whistle-blowing creates dilemmas for both student and qualified nurses alike. One senior nurse advised that when in a difficult situation, it might help to visualize it on the front page of a newspaper – how would it look? Can you justify your action or lack of action? Always remember the network of student support that is available, such as university lecturers and placement coordinators, trust staff, mentors and managers, peer group support and telephone advice lines run by the NMC and RCN. There is a wealth of experienced people who will be only too happy to offer support and advice. Sometimes it just feels better to talk to someone and air our feelings.

As learning disability nurses do not wear a uniform, it is a good idea to wear clothes that are loose, comfortable and laundry friendly. Trousers and blouses may need to be washed several times a week. One colleague was recently in the wrong place at the wrong time when a client was suffering from projectile vomiting (perhaps this is not the time to mention the diarrhoea he was also suffering from!), so it can also be prudent to have a spare set of clothes nearby, working on the assumption that if you do not have any you will definitely need them! It is probably also a good idea to leave the designer gear at home.

The forensic service

If as a student nurse you are fortunate to be offered the opportunity of a placement in the forensic service, there are some basic guidelines. These include reading unit policies and client care plans – it is important to remember that these clients are offenders and should not be underestimated, however inoffensive or likeable they appear. The wearing of suitable clothes is essential and can be discussed before beginning the placement. No personal information should be discussed with clients or within earshot of clients. This includes any information regarding family members, addresses and especially not photographs. Offenders, particularly sex offenders, can be very manipulative and use the information for their own benefit. Physical contact between fellow staff or clients is also seriously discouraged, this includes hugs and kisses at the end of the placement! But providing the unit advice is followed the placement should be fascinating and a superb learning opportunity.

Helpful books and resources

Useful reading simply has to include *Learning Disabilities* by Gates, which covers a wide range of topics related to learning disabilities, from social policy to genetic disorders. *The A–Z of Syndromes and Inherited Disorders* by Gilbert is an excellent reference book of conditions for nurses in all branches. The white paper *Valuing People* by the Department of Health sets government targets and planning for people with a learning disability. The Mental Health Act 1983 is useful when working with clients who are held under section (although relevant sections may be preferable to the entire act!). *The Psychology of Criminal Conduct* by Blackburn is a fascinating read when working in forensic nursing. The Human Rights Act (1998) is also useful for clients' basic rights. *Nursing Law and Ethics* by Tingle and Cribb is an excellent book for students of all Branches. Details of all these (and other) resources are in the References section at the end of this appendix). Finally, a good nursing dictionary is a must! Another good tip is to buy books that will also be of use to you after qualifying.

Becoming qualified

Perhaps the most important advice is to believe in your ability to complete the nursing course. The high drop-out rate of student nurses, together with the fact that many mature students have not studied academically for several years, can be very daunting. Younger students have the advantage of being more recently in the education system, perhaps studying subjects useful to nursing such as the sciences, but mature students have the advantage of life experience and time management skills. These different skills are equally important and can be very levelling. From experience, it is not always the brightest students who pass modules but those who have the commitment and determination to succeed and work diligently. The course is a 3-year marathon and not a quick sprint! There are always some students on the course who gain impressive marks when revising for an exam or writing an assignment only days before the submission date, only to become complacent and fail modules at a later date. From experience, these are often the students who later struggle to complete the course, because under-estimated course modules mounted up. Take time and effort to work studiously, prepare and revise while the subject is still fresh in your mind, but only do it once! Try to avoid re-sitting exams or having to re-submit assignments several months after the original deadline.

To some students, the thought of being organized is a very unpleasant one. Be organized in writing assignments; even if you work better under pressure and prefer to write assignments close to the submission date, you can carry out research and identify articles needed in advance. For those who, like the writer, are techno-phobes and believe that computers have the ability to plan and sabotage work, please remember that computers only crash or run out of ink on the eve of a deadline. This behaviour is almost unheard of with a month to go!

One student was heard to complain that she very unfairly had three assignment deadlines within 3 days of each other. However, when she was reminded that the assignments had all been launched 6 or 7 months previously she simply answered 'That's not the point'. Being organized, although a very boring concept, also allows for the unexpected, such as a bout of flu or unexpected family commitments. One piece of advice from a lecturer was to type an assignment and 'let it go cold' for a few days, after which it can be proofread objectively and the writer does not read what he or she expects to read.

Never be embarrassed to ask questions in lectures. Many students are just too self-conscious to ask a question or admit they don't understand something in front of so many other people. However, one thing for certain is that there will be many other people who don't know the answer either and are waiting patiently for someone else to ask.

Take advantage of all learning opportunities. The advantages of attending extra sessions such as academic writing groups, skills practice or a day with a paramedic far outweigh having a little extra time off. The 3-year training period is also an ideal opportunity to request placements with different health trusts and in specialist areas, enabling the student nurses to have an overview of how different trusts work. This can also be an opportunity to network, make valuable friendships and learn about career opportunities.

Finally, perhaps the most important and valuable piece of advice any student nurse can have is simply to enjoy the entire experience!

REFERENCES AND BIBLIOGRAPHY

Barton R 1960 Institutional neurosis. Reprinted in: Gates B (ed) 1997 Learning disabilities, 3rd edn. Churchill Livingstone, New York

Blackburn R 1993 The psychology of criminal conduct. John Wiley & Sons, Chichester

Butler B March 2003 Nursing in the 21st century. Learning Disability Practice 6(2): 28

Craft A 1994 Practice issues in sexuality and learning disabilities. Routledge, London

Department of Health 2001 Valuing people: a new strategy for learning disability for the 21st century. The Stationary Office, London

Department of Health 1998 Signposts for success in commissioning and providing health services for people with learning disabilities, NHS Executive, Leeds

Department of Health 1983 Mental health act 1983. DoH, London

Gates B (ed) 1997 Learning disabilities, 3rd edn. Churchill Livingstone, New York

Gilbert P 2000 A–Z of syndromes and inherited disorders, 3rd edn. Stanley Thornes, Cheltenham

Plougher J 1997 Providing quality care. In: Gates B (ed) 1997 Learning disabilities. Churchill Livingstone, New York

Scull A T 1982 Museums of madness. Penguin, Harmondsworth, Middlesex

Swann C 1997 Development of services. In: Gates B (ed) 1997 Learning disabilities. Churchill Livingstone, New York

Tingle J, Cribb A (eds) 1995 Nursing law and ethics. Blackwell Science, Oxford

United Nations (December, 1971) Declaration of rights of mentally retarded persons. United Nations, New York

Wolfensburger W 1972 Cited in Stalker K, Campbell V 1998 Person-centred planning: an evaluation of a training programme. Health and Social Care in the Community 6(2): 130–134

Websites

Learning disabilities: www.learningdisabilitiesuk.org.uk/
Nursing and Midwifery Council: www.nmc-uk.org

Tips for Children's Nursing

These tips come from a discussion with Elaine Elwell, RN, RSCN, District Nurse, BSc (Hons). They are the top ten things Elaine suggests for student children's nurses to bear in mind:

1. Children are not miniature adults; they are special people with specific needs.

2. Children react very quickly, both to illness and to treatment. A child's condition can change very quickly, so you need to be attentive.

3. Parents are usually the single most important people in that child's life – if you don't involve them, you are not being holistic. It's *essential* to involve parents in the care of their child. It's also important to help a child become independent – even a very young child is capable of more than you imagine!

4. Don't ever tell a child a lie, even a little one. You won't easily get trust back once it is lost. Ask permission before touching them and explain things as you do them. Remember that even a child can refuse to give consent.

5. Good boundaries are essential in children's nursing. You need to love the children you care for, but you can't compromise your objectivity and professionalism.

6. Medication administration is very specific in children's nursing – have the necessary formulas and titrations written down and always use them. Children have what is called a 'paradoxical reaction' to many medications – that means that what can make an adult tired can make a child hyperactive and vice versa! Always know what the medication you are giving will do to a *child*.

7. Speak at the appropriate level. Use words a child can understand even if it seems silly. Asking a child if they have opened

their bowels may be confusing – it's better to say, 'Did you poo?' Remember that they will see you as an adult in authority and might need to be given permission to ask questions or express their concerns. It also helps to know what trends are current in children's TV and books so you have something to talk about!

8. Children use a lot of non-verbal communication. When caring for children, you need to be sensitive to what they *don't* say, and how they behave. Just because a child is quiet or sleeping doesn't mean they aren't in pain or very ill. Don't take anything for granted.

9. Children are insightful and have a way of knowing things you don't expect them to. They might not tell you they know because they are trying to protect *you*! Honest communication is important, but never lead anyone to lose hope.

10. As a children's nurse you will have heartache and tears but you will also have joy and satisfaction. Take care of yourself: you can't take care of anyone else if you don't take care of yourself.

Normal Values

BLOOD (HAEMATOLOGY)

Test	Reference range
Activated partial thromboplastin time (APTT)	30–40 s
Bleeding time (Ivy)	2–8 min
Erythrocyte sedimentation rate (ESR)	
Adult women	3–15 mm/h
Adult men	1–10 mm/h
Fibrinogen	1.5–4.0 g/L
Folate (serum)	4–18 µg/L
Haemoglobin	
Women	115–165 g/L
	(11.5–16.5 g/dL)
Men	130–180 g/L (13–18 g/dL)
Haptoglobins	0.3–2.0 g/L
Mean cell haemoglobin (MCH)	27–32 pg
Mean cell haemoglobin concentration (MCHC)	30–35 g/dL
Mean cell volume (MCV)	78–95 fL
Packed cell volume (PCV or haematrocrit)	
Women	0.35–0.47 (35–47%)
Men	0.40–0.54 (40–54%)
Platelets (thrombocytes)	150–400×10^9/L
Prothrombin time	12–16 s
Red cells (erythrocytes)	
Women	3.8–5.3×10^{12}/L
Men	4.5–6.5×10^{12}/L
Reticulocytes (newly formed red cells in adults)	25–85×10^9/L
White cells total (leucocytes)	4.0–11.0×10^9/L

BLOOD – VENOUS PLASMA (BIOCHEMISTRY)

Test	Reference range
Alanine aminotransferase (ALT)	10–40 U/L
Albumin	36–47 g/L
Alkaline phosphatase	40–125 U/L
Amylase	90–300 U/L
Aspartate aminotransferase (AST)	10–35 U/L
Bicarbonate (arterial)	22–28 mmol/L
Bilirubin (total)	2–17 μmol/L
Caeruloplasmin	150–600 mg/L
Calcium	2.1–2.6 mmol/L
Chloride	95–105 mmol/L
Cholesterol (total)	ideally below 5.2 mmol/L
HDL-cholesterol	
Women	0.6–1.9 mmol/L
Men	0.5–1.6 mmol/L
$PaCO_2$ (arterial)	4.4–6.1 kPa
Copper	13–24 μmol/L
Cortisol (at 08.00 h)	160–565 nmol/L
Creatine kinase (total)	
Women	30–150 U/L
Men	30–200 U/L
Creatinine	55–150 μmol/L
Gamma-glutamyl transferase (γGT)	
Women	5–35 U/L
Men	10–55 U/L
Globulins	24–37 g/L
Glucose (venous blood, fasting)	3.6–5.8 mmol/L
Glycosylated haemoglobin (HbA$_1$)	4.0–6.5%
Hydrogen ion concentration (arterial)	35–44 nmol/L

(continued)

Test	Reference range
Iron	
Women	10–28 μmol/L
Men	14–32 μmol/L
Iron-binding capacity total (TIBC)	45–70 μmol/L
Lactate (arterial)	0.3–1.4 mmol/L
Lactate dehydrogenase (total)	230–460 U/L
Lead (adults, whole blood)	<1.7 μmol/L
Magnesium	0.7–1.0 mmol/L
Osmolality	275–290 mmol/kg
PaO_2 (arterial)	12–15 kPa
Oxygen saturation (arterial)	>97%
pH	7.36–7.42
Phosphate (fasting)	0.8–1.4 mmol/L
Potassium (serum)	3.6–5.0 mmol/L
Protein (total)	60–80 g/L
Sodium	136–145 mmol/L
Transferrin	2–4 g/L
Triglycerides (fasting)	0.6–1.8 mmol/L
Urate	
Women	0.12–0.36 mmol/L
Men	0.12–0.42 mmol/L
Urea	2.5–6.5 mmol/L
Uric acid	
Women	0.09–0.36 mmol/L
Men	0.1–0.45 mmol/L
Vitamin A	0.7–3.5 μmol/L
Vitamin C	23–57 μmol/L
Zinc	11–22 μmol/L

CEREBROSPINAL FLUID

Test	Reference range
Cells	0–5 mm^3
Chloride	120–170 mmol/L
Glucose	2.5–4.0 mmol/L
Pressure (adult)	50–180 mm/H$_2$0
Protein	100–400 mg/L

URINE

Test	Reference range
Albumin/creatinine ratio	<3.5 mg albumin/mmol creatinine
Calcium (diet dependent)	<12 mmol/24 h (normal diet)
Copper	0.2–0.6 μmol/24 h
Cortisol	9–50 μmol/24 h
Creatinine	9–17 mmol/24 h
5-Hydroxyindole-3-acetic acid (5HIAA)	10–45 μmol/24 h
Magnesium	3.3–5.0 mmol/24 h
Oxalate	
Women	40–320 mmol/24 h
Men	80–490 mmol/24 h
pH	4–8
Phosphate	15–50 mmol/24 h
Porphyrins (total)	90–370 nmol/24 h
Potassium (depends on intake)	25–100 mmol/24 h
Protein (total)	no more than 0.3 g/L
Sodium (depends on intake)	100–200 mmol/24 h
Urea	170–500 mmol/24 h

FAECES

Test	Reference range
Fat content (daily output on normal diet)	<7 g/24 h
Fat (as stearic acid)	11–18 mmol/24 h

Agenda for Change

By the time you read this, Agenda for Change (AFC) should be either a reality or pretty close. This appendix is intended just to briefly explain what AFC is, what came before and what AFC means for nursing.

Before there was AFC, there was the Whitley Council Clinical Grading. In 1988 nursing was given an overhaul. Nurses were broken down into a number of categories, from D to I. Although there was guidance for staff and management, there were countless appeals and after time it was felt that clinical grading was not a fair and appropriate career progression system for nurses. Under this system, a 'D'-grade nurse who wanted to advance had to look for an 'E'-grade post – there was no natural progression with time and experience. To get into higher pay bands, nurses needed to leave bedside nursing and go into management roles. Also, nurses with experience in one area started back at the bottom if they moved somewhere else:

> I feel like being a 'D' grade is a terminal illness – there hasn't been an 'E' grade opening on this ward for years ... it's not fair. I love nursing and I love the kinds of patients I have here but I am not getting credit for my skills and experience ... I feel like the 'D' is the scarlet letter!
>
> *Nurse who had spent 7 years as a D grade*

> It's not a fair system. I have the same kinds of responsibilities as some nurses but I am paid much less... it should be similar pay for similar work.
>
> *Physiotherapy team leader*

AFC was developed in response to complaints like these and lobbying from pressure groups and unions representing employees all over the NHS. Key points in AFC are that it:

- puts all NHS employees, with the exception of doctors, dentists and senior managers, into two pay spines (one for pay review body (PRB) staff, one for non-PRB staff)
- seeks to equalize similar work with similar pay
- seeks to equalize conditions and hours
- uses bands rather than Whitley grades
- places roles into bands based on job evaluations
- bases the job evaluations on 16 factors
- enables pay progression through 'steps' in the band
- assesses employees at the gateways to new steps
- bases assessment on knowledge and skills framework that is harmonized with the job evaluation process.

This means that nurses will have:

- The ability to progress in pay without having to change jobs or leave direct patient care nursing.
- A sensible equal equal-pay-for-equal-work system where everyone in the NHS is paid within a similar structure.
- Assessment of knowledge and skills and support for training and development (knowledge and skills framework).

Every job in the NHS will be evaluated based on a number of factors:

1. communication and relationship skills
2. knowledge, training and experience
3. analytical skills
4. planning and organizational skills
5. physical skills
6. responsibility – patient/client care
7. responsibility – policy and service delivery
8. responsibility – financial and physical assets
9. responsibility – human resources
10. responsibility – information resources

11. responsibility – research
12. freedom to act (authority)
13. physical effort
14. mental effort
15. emotional effort
16. working conditions (including exposure to risk and hazards).

Each factor is broken down into different levels. The level at which a particular factor is weighted for a particular job is calculated (for example, a nurse will have greater expectations in the area of patient care than a painter will) and is given a score. These scores are added up, and the job is placed into a pay band based on the overall score. The pay bands are in a number of steps.

A knowledge and skills framework (KSF) will outline the necessary skills for each particular job. The person in a specific job will be able to see clearly what he or she is expected to do in that job. It is anticipated that employees and management will work together both to assess the individual and to plan for opportunities to grow and develop in the job role.

As a person progresses through a particular pay band, he or she will need to demonstrate that he or she has met the expectations for the position they hold. If there are deficits (for example, if the knowledge and skills framework and the job description specify that a nurse needs to learn phlebotomy and hasn't), then the person could be held back at his or her current pay step. However, it is the responsibility of management to offer the employee opportunities to gain the knowledge and skills needed. If the nurse has applied for the phlebotomy course numerous times but wasn't able to go because of staffing levels, that nurse might argue that he or she has not been given the chance and, as a result, should not be penalized. Advancement and achievement are seen as the responsibility both of the employee and the NHS.

Just as there were grievances and appeals when clinical grading was put into place, so there will be issues when AFC is put into place (hopefully) in October 2004. However, most of those involved in the process of planning and implementing the process believe that it is a fair and sensible system that offers good pay and career progression, fairness and equity in pay, a way to assess and maintain skills and knowledge, and support for training and development.

Some of the differences between clinical grading and AFC are:

- AFC has one set of rules for employees and employers (clinical grading had different rules for different parties – employers, employees and NHS management).
- AFC is being piloted (April 2003 to 2004) and elements will be re-assessed after the pilot; clinical grading was put into place without piloting or review.
- AFC is across the board for all NHS staff (except doctors and consultants).
- AFC was preceded by a long period of consultation, negotiation and discussion with representatives from staff all over the NHS.
- There is clear and easily accessible guidance for the criteria for each job in the NHS under AFC.
- There is a difference in the way unsocial hours will be paid.

Visit the DoH website (www.doh.gov.uk) and search for Agenda for Change – it will give you the most current information and publications available.

This has been a very basic explanation of AFC but I hope it helps you understand what all the fuss is about! Whether you are a newly qualified D-grade staff nurse or a band 6 nurse, remember that even though you are there to take care of patients, you have to take care of yourself, too. Having fair pay and working conditions is essential if you are expecting to give your best for the people for whom you care.

Root words, Prefixes and Suffixes

ROOT WORDS

Root word	Meaning
acou	hearing
acr	extremities, height
aden	gland
aer	air
algesi	pain
andr	male
angi	vessel, duct
angi	vessel
ankyl	crooked, stiff, bent
arter	artery
arthr	joint
articul	joint
atel	imperfect, incomplete
ather	yellowish, fatty plaque
aur	ear
aut	self
axill	armpit
bil	bile
blast	developing cell
blephar	eyelid
brachi	arm
bronch	bronchus
bucc	cheek
cancer	cancer
carcin	cancer
cardi, coron	heart
caud	tail

(*continued*)

Root word	Meaning
celi	abdomen
ceph, cephal	head
cerv	neck (like neck of a bottle)
cheil	lip
chole	gall, bile
chondr	cartilage
chrom	color
cortic	outer layer of an organ
cost	rib
crani	head
crani	skull
cry	cold
crypt	hidden
cutane	skin
cyan	blue
cyst	bladder, sac
cyt, cyte	cell
cyte	cell
dacry	tear, tear duct
dactyl	fingers or toes
dent	tooth
derm	skin
dermat	skin
dextr	right
dipl	double
dips	thirst
dynam	power or strength
ectop	located away from usual place
electr	electricity, electrical activity
encephal	brain
entera	entrails (guts)
esthesi	sensation, feeling
eti	cause (of disease)
faci	face, covering
gastr	stomach
gloss	tongue
gluc	sweetness; sugar
glycos	sugar
gynae	woman
haem	blood

Root word	Meaning
hepa, hepat	liver
heter	other
hist	tissue
homo	same, unchanging
hydr	water
hypn	sleep
irid	iris
isch	deficiency
kal	potassium
kerat	hard tissue
kinesi	motion, movement
labi	lips
lacrim	tears, tear duct
lact	milk
lapar	abdomen
later	side
leuk	white
lingu	tongue
lip	fat
lith	stone
mamm, mast	breast
mandibu	lower jaw
maxil	upper jaw
meatus	opening
melan	black
ment	mind, thinking
metr	uterus
mono	one
morph	form
my, myos	muscle
myc	fungus
myel	bone marrow, spinal cord
myelon	bone marrow
myo, musculo	muscle
myring	eardrum
nas	nose
nat	birth
necr	death, dead

(*continued*)

Root word	Meaning
nephr, ren	kidney
neur	nerve
neuro	nerve
noct	night
ocu	eye
olig	few
onc	tumor
onych	nail
oo, ov	egg; ovum
ophth	vision, the eye
orch, orchid	testis, testicle
orth	straight
oste	bone
ot	ear
ox	oxygen
pachy	thick
part	birth
path	disease
pector	chest
pelv	pelvis, pelvic bone
phag	eat, swallow
phas	speech
phleb	vein
phot	light
phren	mind
plasm	plasma, in the blood
pneumo, pnea	air, lung
pod	foot
poster	back (of body)
pseud	fake; false
psych	mind
py	pus
pyr	fever, heat
quadr	four
rhin	nose
sarc	flesh, connective tissue
scoli	crooked, curved
sept	septum
septum	division, wall

Root word	Meaning
sinus	empty space
som	the body
somat	body
somn	sleep
spir	breath
spir	breathe, breathing
splen	spleen
spondyl	spine or vertebrae
spondyl	vertebra, spinal or vertebral column
stoma	mouth, an opening
therm	heat
thorac	thorax (chest)
thromb	clot
tom	cut, section
top	place, outside
tymp	drum
ungu	nail
ure, uri	urine
vas	vascular, veins, duct
vesi-	pouch, sac

PREFIXES

Prefix	Meaning
a-, an-	without, missing
ab-	from, away from
ad-	to, toward
ambi-	both
ante-	before
anti-	against
bi-, bin-	two
brady-	slow
chlor-	green
circum-	around
cirh-	yellow

(continued)

Prefix	Meaning
con-	together
contra-	against
cyan-	blue
de-	take way, reduce
dia-	complete
dis-	undo, take away from
dys-	difficult, abnormal
ecto-	outside
endo-	inside
epi-	on, over, covering
erythr-	red
eu-	normal, good
ex-, exo-	outside
extra-	outside of
glauc-	gray
hemi-	half
hetero-	different
homo-	same
hyper-	above, in excess
hypo-	below, deficient
in-, im-	not,
infra-	underneath, below
inter-	between
intra-	inside
jaun-	yellow
leuk/o-, leuc/o-	white
macro-	large
mal-	bad, abnormal
melan-	black
meso-	middle, medium
meta-	change
micro-	small
mono-	one
multi-	many
neo-	new
pan-	all
para-	next to, around, beyond
per-	through
peri-	surrounding

Prefix	Meaning
poly-	many
post-	after
pre-, pro-	before
pseudo-	fake
purpur-	purple
quad-	four
re-	back, again
retro-	behind
rube-	red
semi-	half
sub-	under, beneath
super-, supra-	over, above
sym-, syn-	together, joined
tachy-	fast
trans-	through, across
tri-	three
ultra-	above, beyond, extra
uni-	one

SUFFIXES

Suffix	Meaning
-aemia, -emia	blood
-algia	pain
-cele	hernia
-centesis	tap, puncture
-clasis	to break down
-desis	binding, stabilization
-dynia	pain, swelling, discomfort
-ectasis	dilation, expansion
-ectomy	removal
-gen	beginning
-gram	record of data
-graph	instrument for recording

(continued)

Suffix	Meaning
-graphy	act of recording data
-ia	an unhealthy state
-iac	indicates person has certain conditions
-iasis	abnormal condition, presence of
-icle	small
-ism	condition, state of being
-ist	a specialist
-itis	inflammation
-lysis	loosen, destruction
-malacia	softening
-megaly	enlargement
-meter	instrument for measuring
-metry	measurement of
-oid	resemble
-ole	small
-oma	tumour, swelling
-osis	abnormal condition
-pathy	disease
-penia	decrease, deficiency
-pexy	fixation, suspension
-phagia	eating, swallowing
-phasia	speech
-phobia	fear
-plasty	formation, repair
-plegia	paralysis
-ptosis	prolapse, drooping
-rrhage	burst forth
-rrhapy	suture
-rrhea	discharge
-rrhexis	rupture
-sclerosis	hardening
-scope	instrument for viewing
-scopy	examination
-spasm	involuntary contraction, twitching
-stomy	forming an opening
-tomy	incision, to cut into
-tripsy	to crush
-ule	small
-y	condition, process

These are special suffixes that show singular and plural endings.

Singular	Plural
-a	ae
-ax	aces
-en	ina
-ix/-ex	ices
-sis	ses
-on	a
-um	a
-us	i
-y	ies
-ma	mata

REFERENCES

Cohen B 1998 Medical terminology – an illustrated guide. Lippincott-Raven Publishers, Philadelphia

Gyls B, Wedding M 1983 Medical terminology: a systems approach. FA Davis, Philadelphia

Nurse Prescribing

❛ It never made sense – any time I went to the GP to ask for wound-care products, she always asked me what I wanted and gave it to me without even asking about the patient. When the GP needs to prescribe dressings for other patients, they call and ask the district nurses what would be best. All that nurse prescribing has done is cut out the time to consult the GP, who doesn't really know about wound care anyway ... ❜

District Nurse, Nurse Prescriber

CONTEXT

Nurse prescribing started in 1986 when the Cumberlege Report recommended allowing certain groups of nurses (district nurses and health visitors) to prescribe certain medications and products. Other government reports followed, making similar recommendations. There was tremendous resistance – it took 6 years just to get the legislative changes needed to pilot nurse prescribing. It then took a number of years – and a tremendous amount of work – to convince the government (and the British Medical Association!) that nurses could be safe, competent and reliable prescribers. Starting in 1992, there were numerous pilot studies that, even though from the very beginning, were successful but which were repeated until it could be plainly seen that their success was the norm rather than a quirk. Nurses faced opposition because the medical community and pharmacists felt that nurses lacked the necessary diagnostic and assessment skills to prescribe safely, and lacked understanding of pharmacodynamics and the usage of medications. Nurses had to prove beyond doubt that they were expert in their specific area of practice and could competently and safely prescribe before nurse prescribing could become a reality.

Nurse prescribing offers a number of benefits to the healthcare team and to the patient. Some of these benefits are:

- no waiting for a GP – saves GP, patient and nurse time
- products are being prescribed by the person actually doing the patient care
- opportunities for nurse innovation and nurse-led clinics
- patients feel that they can talk to nurses, and feel that nurses are approachable and accessible.

WHO ARE NURSE PRESCRIBERS?

There are currently two levels of nurse prescriber:

1. **The independent prescriber:** this nurse can make decisions about the patients and their needs and prescribe from a limited formulary without consulting a doctor. This nurse is responsible for making the correct diagnosis and developing the appropriate treatment plan.

2. **The supplementary prescriber:** this nurse can prescribe for certain illnesses for which there is an agreed protocol, or can follow-up treatment after the patient has been diagnosed by a doctor.

A subset of the *British National Formulary* (BNF) – the nurse prescriber's formulary (NPF) – lists the items a nurse can prescribe. A companion book called the *Drug Tariff* explains the packaging and prices for items in the BNF/NPF.

Most commonly, district nurses, health visitors and practice nurses are independent prescribers. These, and other nurses who offer care to specific groups of patients, for example a practice nurse running an asthma clinic, can train for extended prescribing privileges so that they can offer more comprehensive and coordinated care. Extended prescribing is intended for patients with minor injuries and minor ailments, those needing palliative care and for health promotion.

As this is being written, nurses all over the UK are looking for opportunities to innovate and transform the way care is delivered in both primary (community) and secondary (hospital) settings. The government has recognized this and is actively looking at nurse prescribing and how the role of the nurse is changing.

In April 2002, Alan Milburn (at that time the Secretary of State for Health), announced at the RCN Congress:

> ❛ I have asked the CNO to work with the Nursing and Midwifery Council and higher education to review and reform nurse pre-registration training so that in future nurse prescribing can be enshrined in the training of every single newly qualified nurse. ❜

Although nothing has yet been put into place, the reality is that pre-registration nurse education will include at least basic nurse prescribing at some point in the future.

Because it is not yet known what kind of formulary (list of medications) would be used for newly qualified nurses and because nurse prescribing in general is evolving rapidly, this appendix won't discuss the different medications and appliances that nurses prescribe. What I can give you is information about where to find out more and a framework for decision making used by nurse prescribers. Chapter 8 contains the complete NMC *Guidelines for the Administration of Medicines,* and when prescribing these must still be followed.

'OK, I don't know what I will be able to prescribe, or when, but when I do …' As in any part of nursing, the way you make decisions is key to proving that your decisions are competent and appropriate. The prescribing pyramid is a framework for responsible decision making from the National Prescribing Centre.

SEVEN PRINCIPLES OF GOOD PRESCRIBING

1. Examine the holistic needs of the patient. Is a prescription necessary?
2. Consider the appropriate strategy.
3. Consider the choice of product.

4. Negotiate a 'contract' and achieve concordance with the patient.
5. Review the patient on a regular basis.
6. Ensure record keeping is both accurate and up to date.
7. Reflect on your prescribing.
    (NPC 1999)

1. Examine the holistic needs of the patient

What are the patient's needs? Are there some products that are inappropriate because of cultural, religious or personal values or beliefs? For example, some medications are made with animal products and so are not suitable for vegetarians. The only way to be sure is to make a good holistic assessment of the patient.

2. Consider the appropriate strategy

What are you trying to accomplish? What is your goal in treating this patient? What is the evidence you are using to make your decision? What alternatives are there?

3. Consider the choice of product

Does the patient have allergies? What is the cost effectiveness of this product? How is it used? Does it have any side-effects or interactions? Is it in accordance with your strategy and your assessment?

4. Patient concordance

Have you discussed your strategy with the patient? Does he or she agree? Will he or she comply with the medication regimen? Does he or she understand the need to use this product? Does he or she know what possible side-effects or problems to expect and what to do if any occur?

5. Review the patient on a regular basis

Is the product still appropriate? Has it worked? If not, how does that affect the patient and the patient's outcomes? What needs to change? Why didn't it work? If it did work, did it work well enough? How does the patient feel? Does the patient believe he or she still needs this product? Are there any side-effects or problems? You will need to do another assessment of the patient.

6. Record keeping

Records must be accurate and up to date. You must follow all the guidelines for records and record keeping; in addition, there will be special guidelines for the process through which you prescribe.

7. Reflect

How did you make the decisions you made? Were they the right ones? What evidence did you use? Looking back, what would you do differently? Did you really meet the patient's needs? What additional information or knowledge would you need in the future?

If you go through each of these steps, you are showing that you are making responsible and informed decisions about your patients and their care.

It won't be long before nurses are prescribing more items – and pharmacists too will have authority to prescribe. Understanding your role as a nurse and the decision-making framework to make

safe, competent and appropriate decisions will be a good foundation
for you as a potential nurse prescriber.

RECOMMENDED RESOURCES

Two very useful websites have more information about nurse prescribing:

The Department of Health website nurse prescribing page: www.doh.gov.
   uk/nurseprescribing/index.htm
National Prescribing Centre: www.npc.co.uk/
National Prescribing Centre 1999 Prescribing pyramid/seven principles of
   good prescribing. Prescribing Nurse Bulletin 1(1)

A couple of good books are:

Humphries J, Green J (eds) 1999 Nurse prescribing. Palgrave, London
Luker K, Wolfson D 1999 Medicines management for clinical nurses.
   Blackwell Science, Oxford

Other publications:

The *British National Formulary/Nurse Prescriber's Formulary* and the
   Drug Tariff are very useful – ask a pharmacist or a community nurse
   about them.
The *Nursing Standard, Nursing Times, Journal of Advanced Nursing and the
   British Journal of Community Nursing's 'Nurse Prescribing'* all have
   information and resources about nurse prescribing.

Index